Alone On The Yellow Brick Road

A Memoir

On Love, Life, Death, Grief, and Moving On

Beverly Kalinin

Alone On The Yellow Brick Road
A Memoir

ISBN: 978-1-935125-40-2

Book printed in the United States of America

To order additional copies of this book go to:

www.rp-author.com/Kalinin

Beverly Kalinin is available for Readings and Workshops.
She can be reached at: beverlykalinin@sbcglobal.net

Robertson Publishing
59 N. Santa Cruz Avenue, Suite B
Los Gatos, California 95030 USA
(888) 354-5957 · www.RobertsonPublishing.com

Dedicated to my dear Bob over the rainbow

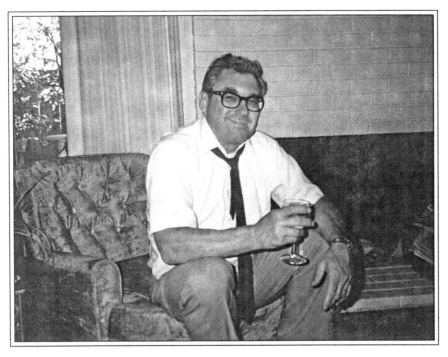

"It's the greatest day of my entire life!" —Bob Kalinin

Acknowledgments

I am deeply grateful to Evelyn Pine, Susan Gold, and Patsy Fergusson, my loving sister writers, whose constant support and encouragement helped me launch this book, finally.

Also, I wish to thank the many friends and relatives that, during the nine months of Bob's illness, kept in touch with him and with me through phone calls, emails, letters, and prayers.

Throughout many of the weeks during that time my dear friends, Tish Matulich, Carol Cameron, and Louise Simson provided us with dinners delivered to our door. I thank them for their kindness.

To my daughter, Judi, I say thank you as well for your gentle nurturing of your father and for the emotional and physical support you gave me.

I am glad, too, that my little Alaskan band—my older daughter, Star, and granddaughters, Sienna and Terra—were here with Bob in his last days.

I extend a special thank you to the Redwood City Kaiser Hospital Hospice team of nurses, aids, social workers, and respite helpers. They gave generously of themselves. They are angels.

Without the folks in my two grief support groups at Kaiser Redwood City and Mills Hospital in San Mateo I would have suffered even more than I have done. Thank you to them and to our leaders Evie Dwyer and Mary Moray.

Thank you, all my sweet friends, near and far, who, with me and my girls honored Bob's life at his Memorial Celebration in San Mateo on August 19, 2005.

Finally, thank you, friends, who continue to be there for me now.

Foreword

They say one dies as he has lived. Likewise, how we have lived is how we will grieve. This is the main theme of *Alone on the Yellow Brick Road*, which is more than a book on grieving. As well, it is a love story.

In the months following the death of my husband of fifty years I attended support groups where, listening to others, I perceived emerging patterns of their grieving processes. With time I determined these patterns of healing were based on how the people had handled other problems in their lives. Generally, the degree of success they had had in living positively and well was consistent with how they dealt with grief. Finally, I decided that the history, spirit, and quality of one's life was directly consistent with that of one's mourning process.

Soon, I wondered how this theory applied to me. I decided to list the grief issues I faced. Examining how I had dealt with similar problems in the past would give me insight and tools for working through my process now. For instance, how had I always handled fear, loneliness, dependency versus independence, or sexuality?

To illustrate these issues, I decided to show the incidents of my life, as well as those of Bob's, that accounted for his brave acceptance of dying and my frightened condition in surviving without him. How would I go forth as a widow? What could I expect from the future? And what elements of my life would heal me best?

Probing for answers and seeking to recover from grief found its result in this memoir, *Alone on the Yellow Brick Road*.

Chapter 1

When Bob had been dead four months I thought I had a stranglehold on desperation at last. Rather, it had one on me, for I could not scream. I knew that if I could scream the protective wall of Prozac would crack open. And the wave of grief escaping would not have resembled "magical thinking," as Joan Didion describes her bereavement. Instead, a torrent of emotion could have swept me away with a force more terrible even than the fury of the moods that rendered me manic at times, then later, spent and staring. That was two years ago.

At about that time I dreamed of 203 Gates Street again. I turned the doorbell knob that jangled like an old wind-up toy. "Remember me? I came here before," I said in my dream when the new owner of my godmother's house opened the door. Inside, my beloved Katie, dead many years, left her chore of setting out party crystal to embrace me. But my eyes searched past her and other ghosts for a glimpse of Bob who appeared only in the background of my dreams and never smiling. This time I did not see him at all, though I sensed his presence, so I allowed myself to awaken.

It was six a.m., time to rub arnica gel into my plantar fasciitis. This common heel pain condition started when I was caring for my sick Bob, and I ignored it. The psychic cause for foot ailments is fear of the future. Now I accepted this information as a sign and decided to heal the heel.

As when Bob was ill and we drew from every available form of healing—allopathic, acupuncture, clinical trials, chemotherapy, affirmations, meditation, diet, and pill box full of medications—I, too, used a variety in my heel healing plan. In addition to accepting my doctor's diagnosis of plantar fasciitis and the metaphysical explanation of heal pain, (of course all widows are afraid of the future), I studied the word root. (Interesting word itself, "root," in this context, as our feet root us to this earth, which is home for our bodies and which keeps us connected to and in balance with this life.)

Ten days after Bob's death I had looked it up. The dictionary definition of heel read: 1) close behind, subservient. v. to follow in the heels of, "the dog following the hunter," to heel. My symbolic plantar fasciitis before Bob died was represented in this definition, I decided. I had stayed behind the healing. I had been subservient to it. I had doggedly served the healing. The next definition read: 2) to lean to one side, to cause to lean. With Bob gone, I was heeling. I was off balance, leaning to one side, and twice falling down.

After the arnica application in the morning, I took my inflammation and pain meds. I applied ice and did exercise twice a day. I read the San Francisco Chronicle and, because Bob had paid up the Wall Street Journal for a year, I brought it into the house, too. Some days I drank my coffee on the driveway, glancing at a scarlet sky, sitting on a child's shabby chair left over from my teen granddaughters. Sometimes I cried there. A pink-and-blue-robed grandma sitting on a tiny chair, wearing a bulky red fleece jacket, and maybe a hat, scarf, or gloves

Back in the house, sighing and beginning another day without Bob, I made the day's list of chores. But first I did a little yoga, pleased that I was returning to the practice, comforted by my body's sign to me that after those four months I might be starting back. The list of chores: Go to Redwood City to start up the R.V., drive it around, practice backing up. Get more Death Certificates; do more financial and other paperwork; attend my Grief Support Group. Call the dry rot man; pump the pool after last week's heavy rain because no one wants to service a doughboy swimming pool; and remind my frightened self I can do all these things. Finally, try to scream.

Chapter 2

It is March, 2005, four months <u>before</u> Bob's death. The blood drips at 120 ML per hour, whatever a ML is. I only know it takes three hours for one pint. They call it a unit. He'll have two units this time. We started in early evening. Now dark, the light in his cubicle, enclosed within a circular curtain, is bright enough for me to read and write. Throughout his life Bob liked the light on because, he said, he was afraid of the dark. Only two things ever scared this courageous man, the dark and death.

Mostly he sleeps, occasionally opening his eyes to see if I am there. I am always looking at his face, except once when I fell asleep myself and heard my name and saw his bright eyes at once. He had to pee. We pulled the curtain all the way and he used the plastic urinal. He has to go three times in all, and each time we giggle a little, wondering in whispers where all the pee was when we needed it that afternoon for three hours drinking lattes and much water in the lab waiting room.

The room in shadow beyond our spotlighted bed and chair area reminds me of a darkened theater in which the audience has failed to turn off their electrical devices. At least the television is very low, not like once when his roommate blasted the sound all night, rousing in me a level of anxiety made worse by the thought that Bob was having nine hours of blood poured into him that time as he slept. And the phone of the third person in this room has rung only twice. Bob has dropped off again.

I make a list of new issues to research. How will I keep him from falling? Who will pick him up if he does fall? How will I avoid hurting myself? Will I need respite help, finally, to leave the house? Maybe consider taking that caregiver course. Explore herbalist or acupuncturist for the anemia while remaining on the clinical trial still. Make the bone scan appointment after revisiting the directive with the doctor. Boils down to keywords: <u>walker</u>, <u>shower bar</u>, <u>caregiver</u>, <u>respite</u>.

Now his mouth is open. Two hours more. He is sleeping harder. Good, because his afternoon naps, extended to four and a half hours lately, alarm me. So many of his twenty-four spent vaguely unconscious. The nurse adjusts the machine; it beeps a shrill warning. She stretches the thin red tube; it's dark, almost black. Bob had joked earlier that he hoped this donor was a word jumble whiz. Bob had always been so fast at the word puzzles before. The nurse asked if I wanted coffee for driving home. Not necessary, my adrenalin always races getting his unsteady self home in the wee hours, the parking lot quiet and still, lighted here and there by greenish glows.

We never stay all night. They are always amazed we do not, the nurses and aids. Bob never removes his clothes either, which also surprises them when they offer a hospital gown. He lets me take off his shoes. We just want to rush back to the safe haven of our own home and wake up in our own bed, side by side, with the cat snuggled up, fifty years of different cats and dogs. Snuggled up side by side for fifty years in four and a half months from now.

The collapsed, blood-coated plastic bag, nearly empty, looks vile rather than life giving. An hour left. Later, when we reach home exhausted and open the front door, Dorothy will come meowing down the hallway. Bright and inquiring, she will study each of us in turn. Having scarcely left Bob's side these days, she, no doubt, will be relieved to see him returned intact.

Chapter 3

For the nine months of his illness I was the devoted advocate for my husband's health. In addition to overseeing the clinical trials and chemotherapy prescribed by his doctor, I dragged him to mind/body workshops, presented him with cancer books to read, and provided affirmation tapes for his daily listening. Together we performed gentle physical exercises to keep up his strength. We turned to restricting sugar in his diet because cancer feeds on sugar. Then we reversed that method and I encouraged him to eat as much of everything as he could, including special drinks I ordered through the mail, because he had lost so much weight. Through it all, as he grew weaker, he continued to have blood transfusions and to visit a variety of doctors including the oncologist, urologist, and the cardiologist, as he had congestive heart failure in the middle of it all which landed him in the hospital for a week. There he stoically continued his walking exercise down the hallways of the ICU, unembarrassed by his catheter bag of blood even when some of the nurses glanced askance at it. (Bob bled from his kidney for weeks on end.) Bob readily tried everything I offered and trusted me completely. But his illness progressed so quickly we could never keep ahead with the healing. He never complained. Much later when I could look back on the large picture of his life, I saw it took him nine months to be born and nine months to die.

When it had become time to bring in a hospital bed to our home, I was ready. Weeks before, I had spent hours making a plan one night lying next to him in our king-size bed. For most of the nights of Bob's illness I had been exhausted by bedtime, dropping off heavily, awakening sharply when he moved in his sleep. I got so that I could empty the mid-night catheter with him barely awake. And when he called "Bev" I would spring out to do what was needed. He never wanted to disturb my sleep but I demanded he call me. "Bev," he'd say, so quietly, so gently. I would be disturbed every night for the rest of my life to hear that again.

But on the night I made the plan, I was wide awake, my mind clear and alert. The timing must be perfect. This bed would go and a twin purchased and ready for delivery at the precise, correct time would be placed next to the hospital bed as soon as it arrived. "People usually use another room for the patient," the hospice nurse suggested on that particular morning she was summonsed to our home because I could no longer lift Bob from our bed.

"No," I answered at once. "Together we can move him to the family room sofa bed where we will sleep together tonight," I said. The nurse, my daughter, Judi, and I managed to get Bob into his wheelchair, for by then he could not stand alone. Then we dismantled the marriage bed. On the same day the twin was delivered from the store and the hospital bed from the rental place.

I don't know if Bob realized, as I did, that we were in a bed together that night for the last time. I do believe he would have chosen not to acknowledge the fact, for remaining in denial allowed him to continue to believe in our early-on slogan: *together we would beat this*. I carefully said nothing that would in any way weaken his steadfast resolve to get well. Though we would never sleep in the same bed again, nevertheless, I would make a replica of our bed for us.

The next afternoon the hospice nurse returned, and again Judi, she, and I managed to get him into his wheelchair and back down the hallway to his hospital bed in our bedroom. One sunny window wall there lets us gaze with pleasure at flowers in our patio. It was difficult for Bob to be his enthusiastic, positive self now though. Looking out the window he did not smile.

We watched the last movie we saw together in that room, a video from his large collection: the Clint Eastwood spaghetti westerns, Casablanca, the 007 series, the Wizard of Oz. He watched them over and over, those classics, just as he continued to replay his CD favorites: Ray Charles, Dinah Washington, and the 70s oldies. "Not again," I'd say, coming into his room, the walls of which are covered with movie posters, and seeing him sitting contentedly in his beloved lopsided recliner he refused to replace. I used those dear tapes at the memorial I gave for him but I cannot yet listen to them again at home. The movie we watched that afternoon was *My Cousin Vinny*, a good comedy which I hope gave him some small relief from worry.

At that time he began taking his meals in bed, as he was finally unable to get up at all. Bob was a man of few words so it was hard to know what he was thinking. But one day I entered to find him struggling to do leg lifts. "What are you doing?" I asked in alarm, "don't exhaust yourself." With that, he grabbed the railing in an effort to roll over and sit up. He was too weak. "Bob you can't do this." I imagined him sliding to the floor, as he had done three times prior in his illness.

"I have got to keep up my strength so I can get up. I've got to sit in my wheelchair," he claimed, still straining to turn over.

"You can't do this; you are too weak."

He stopped and lay still. I perceived a slight chink in his protective wall of denial.

"You aren't going to use your wheelchair anymore." I felt I was a betrayer. He stared at me with a delicate mixture of anger, fear, trust, hope, pleading, all so subtle I knew we had reached an awful moment. Now we shared the same truth. He remained still and quiet. I sensed resignation, finally, though courage never deserted him and I believe that at that moment he released his life-long fear of death.

"Are you afraid?" I whispered.

"No," he answered decisively, with steady strength in his surrender. I chose to believe he meant it.

Chapter 4

In December, 2004, three months after Bob took ill and was diagnosed with kidney cancer, we were still in shock. We stayed stoic for each other, but sometimes when he was napping and I lay huddled alone on the living room couch I would whisper, "please, please." Then, as always, Tunis would appear to me. Tunis is a large angel with magnificent wings who has been with me for many years. As a wise, patient, and warm entity, she enters my consciousness with silence. She hovers softly

On one particular afternoon during that period, wrapped up on my couch, I cried "help me" in my mind and Tunis appeared. This time she glided about the room, gently fanning her wings to lighten the space. The air opened and I breathed better. I watched from a fetal position, the brown and tan hand-croqueted comforter tucked around my chin. Finally, without speaking, she opened the front door, and then settled into the orange armchair across the room to watch who would enter.

In streaked "High Energy," a dwarf in a top hat. I could not see his face because he spun as fast as a top, around and around, coming so close to me I felt an invisible jolt through my body. I caught my breath. Quickly he spun out the door and was gone. I had never seen him before and I wondered how I knew his name. For a half minute it was quiet and still.

Next came a dainty, slow-moving, tippy-toed fairy, slight of body, blue-gowned, wispy and fragile. "I am the Meter Maid, so you can meter out this energy," she said with precise, distinct words. Seemingly content with her mission, she continued towards the door with her same deliberate steps. I could see she wore ballet slippers.

I felt as if I were in Munchkin land and Tunis was Glinda, the good witch of Oz. Was this because Bob's favorite movie was *The Wizard of Oz*? Bob's collection of Oz memorabilia given him from friends over the years is large and varied, from pens to posters. After he died, I had used Ray Charles' rendition of *Somewhere Over the Rainbow* in the memorial ceremony. After that I heard the song everywhere. Judi, Star, and I hear references to the Wizard of Oz all the time; we like to believe they are little missives from Bob.

Tunis and I waited again. Two traditionally clad clowns with red noses came bouncing in then. One was highly visible, the other in shadow. I said to them, "Clowns are happy and sad, like comedy and tragedy, aren't they."

"Yes," snapped the first one, the one I could see best. He seemed disappointed, as if he were both pleased and upset that I had gotten the message so quickly, that there would be sad times and happy times, that that is the yin and yang of life, and that I would be able to deal with it. Then to change the mood of the room and perhaps reward me for being brave he somehow ordered many clowns to appear. They took the form of balloons with faces, sad and happy, bobbing throughout the room, some near the ceiling, some closer to the floor. As they floated, looking at me, they instructed me, without words, to be light, not just sorrowful. I cannot remember their using the front door to leave; I believe they simply vanished.

"Enough for now," Tunis said. She closed the front door and sat down next to me, gathering me into her wings so that I rested heavily upon her bosom.

"Relax," she whispered. I allowed myself to sink into her and I nearly fell asleep, but she told me it was okay not to. "I know you like being awake better than being asleep," she acknowledged.

Chapter 5

I will never be the same again. Of course not. Not after fifty-five years of this person in my life. (I met Bob at age fifteen, wed at twenty, lost him three days before our fiftieth anniversary.) I do not have another fifty-five years to re-program myself. A psychotherapist, Judy Tatelbaum, wrote a book about grieving called, *You Don't Have to Suffer*. Tatelbaum states her motivation for writing this book was the death of her mother, followed by that of her father and several close friends. Her main theme holds that one accepts these deaths as part of life's hurts and moves on. She had not lost a spouse.

I, too, have experienced the loss of my mother, father, friends, and beloved pets as well. The people who console me also have lost parents, family, friends, and probably pets. But no one knows, unless they have experienced the death of a husband or wife, that there is no similarity between losing a cherished mate and anyone else. What is more, I find it vaguely bewildering that the widows I know are the only ones <u>not</u> offering sympathy. Do they know the unspoken truth, as I have come to learn it, that we <u>do</u> need to suffer? And are they reluctant to join in my suffering when they are having still to deal with their own?

In the early months following Bob's death I fell twice. Bowls and vases slipped from my hands and broke. I was short of breath, over-weight, and out of physical shape. My heel hurt. I had no stamina; I was constantly fatigued. I was a couch potato, nearly comatose for moments or minutes, anxious, more restless than usual. I was non-reading, non-concentrating, fumbling, forgetful, off balance, light-headed, hardly believing at times that Bob was really dead. The only thing I knew for sure was that I needed to acknowledge the suffering, feel it and go through it, or I would not heal.

In one of my support groups a woman asked the facilitator if she has ever met anyone who did not pull out of their grieving. I guess she meant has anyone died or gone crazy from mourning, two possibilities that frighten us all. In our circle that night we sat still while fifteen pairs of sad eyes searched her face for hope. For me her answer validated why I sought connection with other widows and widowers.

"The ones who come to groups," she said, "are on their way to recovery. It is the person who stays alone or ignores the pain that will have trouble or take much longer getting through."

Her statement makes me think of Betty in another group I attended. She came regularly at first and suddenly disappeared. As a young widow she had nursed her sick husband for years. "I will never get over this," she said vehemently each time the group met. I remember the first time I heard her say it. It had been only two months for me and, in retrospect, I see my determined comments in response arose from a place of shock in which I functioned in those days.

I scanned the faces in our circle, waiting for someone to reply to Betty, and when no one did, I said, " Bob had to go but I am still here. And I have a choice to be joyful or miserable the rest of my life. I intend to be as positive as I can and be joyful." It had been four months for Betty, who met my glance with a stern, blank face. Though kind to everyone, she continued to repeat her mantra at every meeting. "I will never get over this"

She was correct—one can never get over the death of a spouse, but hopefully one can get through it. I knew I would never choose to stay alone and ignore the pain. There was no healthy way to avoid the suffering. I needed to embrace it.

Betty stopped coming to group meetings and I wonder if she is making her way through it. I wonder, too, how Joan Didion is doing. Fragile of body, yet staunchly courageous after her husband's sudden and unexpected death, she travels from city to city reading from her yearlong chronicle of grieving. According to her book, *The Year of Magical Thinking*, she did much research to understand his illness and her own particular process of mourning. The reader understands that Didion's shifts between quoting medical explanations and reciting ethereal poetry soothe and sustain her.

As comforted by her book as I was, I was equally puzzled by its title. "Magical" carries for me such a connotation of enchantment that I must consider Joan Didion all the braver for using the word. For there is nothing enchanting and whimsical about her grim determination to witness her husband's autopsy. I was jolted by her daring assertion to do so and the depth of suffering that presses a widow to delve so desperately to understand why, why, why.

I wonder if she has trouble screaming.

Chapter 6

After reading *The Year of Magical Thinking* I was inspired to share my own mourning experience with others. Joan Didion's example had enabled me to believe that I could bring comfort and insight to widows and widowers in the same way that members of my grief groups had supported me. She had spoken to me. "Yes, this is how it feels," I felt her say. I could speak to others as well. After all, I had done so in two previous books. When my children were teenagers and I, too, was struggling with personal growth I chronicled those years in a volume of poetry. When I was forty I began teaching others self-empowerment through improvisational dance, and I wrote a book about those workshops.

In my grief groups I am understood and nurtured by friends there, and I, in turn, believe I enrich them with encouragement. We help each other. Contact with others is a central element in the healing process. I know the basis of my own healing lies in connecting with people. "Let's share this," I want to write, "and we will all thrive once again." Enthusiastically, I began this memoir about losing a spouse. It would be a win-win for us all.

Then I attended a writer's workshop, met a memoirist lecturer, loved her book on writing the new autobiography, thought about how I must improve my fledging account of my grief, and abruptly stopped writing. And, therefore, sharing. I was grieving still, of course. But something had frozen my flow of words and a tap might crack them into chips of ice, which would melt like tears and disappear into the earth.

Tristine Rainier, the memoirist, suggested so many formulas for presenting an autobiography that my simple story of a woman grieving for her spouse seemed flat. I found myself searching for a theme in my bereavement to embroider back and forth through the cloth of Bob's death. I asked myself, what are the issues behind

15

the sadness, the fear behind the grieving? Where is the red thread through my mourning that would give a pattern of behavior to my whole life? And how, then, are my past experiences influencing the way I grieve? Though aspects of our suffering are universal, each case is personal and individual and, therefore, only the tip of the iceberg of one's entire life. Chipping away at this tip can reveal a vast area of issues beneath the surface of suffering and sadness. Are we to work through our grief in the same manner we have handled our other life issues?

It seems that in scraping away the frozen flow of my grief words I had run into some of my lifelong themes. For instance, <u>independence versus dependence</u>, <u>solitude and loneliness</u>, <u>bravery against fear</u>. In considering facing these issues in regard to my grief, I was troubled by a thought, however. Would dissecting my lifetime problems be a disloyal or demeaning way to remember and mourn Bob?

Lucy Grealy, who spent years in treatment for her disfigured face caused by childhood jaw cancer and its cure, wrote a memoir called, *Autobiography of a Face*. At one book reading a fan asked her how she remembered all those details. Ms. Grealy snapped back, "I didn't. I wrote them. I am a writer. This is a work of literature." The large crowd fell silent. Though this young woman had spent most of her life in physical and emotional anguish she was a poet and writer of fiction first. And so she determined to step away and document her story through literary eyes.

My personal dilemma was that I might have been seeking to do the same: create literature from Bob's death and my suffering. I can forgive Joan Didion for doing that.

But for me, I visualize Bob and myself frozen in a waterfall, encircled by whirling words like bits of hail from which there is no escape.

In the last days of Bob's life his temperature rose and he was extremely thirsty but could not swallow well. He motioned that he wanted, not sips from a spoon or a dropper, but gushes of water coursing throughout his body. In my mind, over and over I see him in that distress and I plea for a melting down that would soothingly, thoroughly, and continually drench him through and through.

Chapter 7

Actually, Bob had been frozen there since the early days of his illness. But we could not acknowledge the fact. Instead, I slipped and slid around him, chipping fervently, calling constantly, "we will make it; we will make it." His gentle eyes followed me. He trusted me. We believed in each other, scurrying from doctor to doctor, from treatment into yet another plan of recovery. I moved with uneasy urgency. Until I felt myself losing balance, I refused to consider that had I rescued him from his frozen state I might only have freed us both to skid anyway, down, down past Trial One and Trial Two, past the Interferon dance, the Avastin treatments, the medications and meditations, the visualizations, blood transfusions, walker and wheelchair, past pounds melting from his body, strength streaming from his muscles, until there remained only sheer determination, which was the essence of Bob, until he surrendered that last bit.

I could not save him. It was not my fault he died. I did all I could. I know it; Bob knew it. He forgives me. I believe these words, but when I think them I become leaden and cannot move. There is a picture frozen in my mind of Bob in Alaska clowning for his small granddaughters, standing in the front yard in tank top and shorts, bare feet, arms extended high overhead in a victory pose. The snow falling on him, we giggling from the protected porch, he laughing, invigorated by the cooling, melting snow he loved as I snapped the photo.

Now, I am giving <u>myself</u> time to melt.

And when I melt how will I have changed? I keep seeing me at fifteen. Perhaps I will start there again, at the time of my life when I was suffering from the old wound. I met Bob at fifteen, but he had nothing to do with causing the old wound. In fact, his death helped me to heal it.

February 21, 1950. He was walking me home from school. Was he wearing his block sweater, the one still hanging in my closet, dark blue with two gold arm stripes, the gold J for Jefferson High proudly displayed on front? Maybe. He spotted two brass washers on the ground, picked them up, put them on my finger. "Now we're engaged," he smiled. I have one still, hanging on the tail of a lop-sided clay animal one of our daughters made at seven or so. I don't know how the other one disappeared, but every February 21 is still special to me.

The sharpest pain of the old wound occurred when I transferred high schools away from Jefferson and I was not allowed by my new school to continue college prep classes. I was assigned to business courses on the second floor of the lovely brick building: shorthand and typing. Languages, math, science, and advanced English, which I wanted, were taught on the first floor. (My group-two, average-student consciousness had stopped me from protesting. But really, the wound had been inflicted before then: don't talk back, get good grades, be a good girl, and mind your manners. At three I answered adults with "Fine thank you and how are you?" which my mom said threw people for a loop.)

I was eight, my brother four, visiting family friends with our parents. We had been served a snack and my brother was whining to leave. Being the dutiful big sister I whispered we had just eaten and it was not polite to leave immediately. Whatever words I used and however quietly I spoke them, my father who reprimanded me harshly, misinterpreted them. I knew I had been misunderstood but I was so embarrassed I could not come to my own defense. The people said, "that's okay," which led me to believe the other adults had misheard me also. The mortification I suffered and the injustice of the situation when I was just trying to be the good guest my parents desired me to be caused me to feel completely helpless.

I continued to function as the model child, doing what was expected of me, seldom speaking up, and not questioning. Besides, I did not know the question, and there would not have been anyone around to answer anyhow. I graduated from high school in three and a half years with a lifetime membership in the California Scholarship Federation and I knew there was more for me in the world than typing and shorthand. I also knew I was not destined for college. No one ever expected that of me, least of all myself, but some of my friends were going to junior college.

"You don't need that," my father grumbled behind his newspaper when I presented the subject to him. "You can get a good job."

"Please." I stopped drying the dishes.

"You're going to get married and have kids." By then Bob and I were really engaged. It was 1952. "What do you need college for?" he sputtered.

In the end he allowed me to attend junior college providing I got a job immediately following that time. I saw an advisor and when I had seated myself timidly in her office I said I wanted to take sociology, psychology, philosophy, and advanced English. The office seemed dark and important. I was apologetic and embarrassed when I added in a small voice, "I want to culture myself." Those were the words I used. She gave me a sad little smile but approved completely and set up a program for me. In two years, after having received an AA degree, I interviewed for a secretarial job as I had promised my father I would and was offered the position before I left the building.

"Lou Ann and I want to get an apartment together." This was my next hurdle. Though he was proud of me, nevertheless, my father was Italian and old-fashioned.

"No daughter of mine will leave this house before she is married." But again he compromised and gave me one month, a kind of freedom vacation with Lou Ann. I donned my little hat and white gloves and commuted by train to my job in San Francisco's financial district.

I was not on a path I had picked, just as grieving now is not the road I want to travel.

Bob, being the first child in his family, as I was in mine, was also placed on a path, not of his choice necessarily. (I told Bob one morning many years later, watching him from bed tie his necktie for work, that I pictured him in a green and black lumber jacket, working physically—he had a strong physique and legs—or on a fishing boat in his sleeveless sweatshirt, big boots, and a watch cap, pulling up nets of shiny sea creatures. He liked that.) But as a boy, Bob had been programmed by his parents to attend the University of California for four years. I never ever resented this; it was the 50s and that was right action. (Besides I did finish college myself years later.)

Not only was I not on a track of my own, but I did not know what that tract should be. And most importantly of all, no one had been there ever to tell me to bravely follow my bliss, to not be afraid of failure, to have faith in myself, and to keep trying. In short, no one counseled me on how to succeed. So how will I know if I can survive Bob's death?

For years I was trusted not to fail at the things I did. I was afraid to fail. But not failing does not guarantee succeeding. I was afraid to do that too. Bob trusted me to get him through his cancer and I did not succeed. In my seventy years of life I have learned tools for survival and truths to live by, one of which is that I cannot control every eventuality. My head knows this but my heart feels the sadness of not succeeding in saving Bob.

Bob saved me instead. When he died I faced living alone for the first time in my entire life. I knew I would need to step onto a path of my choice, finally. He left me alone to succeed or fail at making my own way. As I defrost a bit, I search myself for the old wound. I touch my torso; there are no lesions. I skim my arms, tanned and strong; they reach, lift, and hold. My legs are bruise-free; they transport me well. My hands have no cuts; they grasp firmly. My brain fires rapidly with clarity. Only my heart suffers, but that is not the old wound, it's the new one.

I find the old wound nowhere, unless it has settled into my heel for a while longer until I am truly pain free. With my healed heel will my correct path appear? When I melt completely will I succeed in following it? Alone, without Bob? Is that even possible? I do not believe so when I rock myself in crying and wailing, the mucous running from my nose, scarcely noticed and disregarded.

Chapter 8

The nine months of Bob's dying began in October 2004 when he noticed a blood clot in his urine. The only direction possible on a frozen waterfall is down. Our slide had begun but we didn't know it. Was it cancer? In time, his primary care giver confirmed it. "Just a spot," she said. An oncologist and urologist were consulted. Then, "quite a lot," they agreed. Too big for surgery. No cure for kidney cancer. A second opinion. "Let's find a clinical trial," it was decided.

Bob kept losing blood, catheter bags full of it, so much that he had congestive heart failure, the heart of a youngster with congestive heart failure. A week in the hospital. A cardiologist, too, now. Meds for heart. "Shall we treat heart or cancer? We can't decide," they pondered. More bureaucracy. Is there a clinical trial available, I reminded them? "Yes." Then let's go for cancer. "Oh, oh, didn't qualify on a detail." Find another damn trial!

When Bob returned home from the hospital, I sent a kick-ass letter to his oncologist. *No one in this period of advanced medical history should have to wait from October to December before treatment is begun*, I ranted. On his first night home I awoke every time Bob coughed and remained on guard until I drifted off again. I had not realized how frightened I would be. The last time we had slept together that cough had turned to a wheezing and shortness of breath that brought 911 immediately. Now, Bob, home again with his young heart, had seven kinds of heart medicine to ingest daily. From good health to cancer and heart failure. From no meds to seven of them, with more coming. Bob stared at the bottles in shock.

Christmas was strange that year. Bob and I decorated the tree with sadness, each of us, especially me, trying to be cheerful. I took pictures of Bob saying I needed to finish out the roll from a trip. I wonder why I felt compelled to give him an excuse about the film.

He probably didn't believe me anyway. The tree was a seven-foot old-fashioned Douglas Fir laden with fifty years of collected baubles and a thousand tiny colored lights. Our prized relic was a separate string of bigger bulbs dating from our first Christmas in 1955. This string blinked on and off at the slow, gentle rate of an earlier era in time, not like the frantic running lights now that remind me of a gambling casino. It's the first thing to go on the tree and we always reminisce a bit about it—how I bought it on my lunch hour at Owl Drug Store (a long defunct chain) in the financial district of San Francisco. Blinking lights were new and rare and all our friends always enjoyed them in our tiny first apartment, their illumination creating on and off tree-branch designs on the ceiling. Now only a few lights work on our string, years ago replacement bulbs became unavailable. The lighted tree with its one cherished, reliable, antique string and its multitude of colored Asian-made new tiny bulbs, light weight and as flighty as fireflies, cheered me.

But on the second day the tree went dark. I was overcome with sadness. That is, until I became determined to fix it. I can do this, I thought. Carefully I followed the many strings that wound around and throughout the tinseled branches. If I could only find the connection of each string to the next and repair or replace it, just get rid of the bad part and rescue the rest, the good part. Maybe there was just one destroyed light, or at most one malfunctioning string. I would start at one end. I would follow it through. I would be thorough. I would be diligent. I would make the tree come to life again. If I just tried hard enough I could save it. I could do this, I could do it. And I did! I did find the one string. I cut it out and threw it away. I connected the healthy parts and the tree lighted again and was beautiful and full of bright life and promise once more. And I felt strong and confident, relieved and happy. Elated, I just knew the upcoming year would be good, a new year of hope.

The last week of the year became a sinister deadline in which, with anxiety, I felt compelled to do everything at once: take Bob to cancer support group, research cachexia (fast weight loss which he was experiencing), consider sugar free foods, read health and nutrition books with Bob, continue to kick start the doctors about a clinical trial. While I moved fast and yet treaded air, my poor Bob groped through a fog of his own. He could not make up his mind on anything but agreed to everything I proposed. How in the world could I help him, I agonized. And then I knew how, when I heard him break through the fog occasionally with his infectious laughter. I decided to follow the laughter back through the hole to the incident or circumstance that allowed his temporary escape from misery and worry. So each time he laughed I crawled into the tunnel, dragging him with me, to the incident of perpetuated laughter where we were healed for a moment

New Year's Eve, 2004, 7 p.m., the living room. A NPR station is playing quiet jazz. There's a fire in the fireplace, cold white wine in a blue stemmed glass, and two squat Christmas candles glowing on the coffee table. I am on the couch, my legs curled under me, watching the tree. Its restored lights warm my spirits as reassuringly as the moving fire flames soothe my body and soul.

Bob is in his cozy room down the hall, in his recliner, snoozing. He is tired most of the time now. I am waiting for him to awaken for our special steak dinner. I hear the Three Stooges marathon in the background. Bob loves them. Because I know he has been laughing or at least smiling at them, their ridiculous sounds comfort me, as does the rain in the patio. I feel layer upon layer of hope tucking us in safely this night.

Now Shirley Horn is playing the piano and singing, *Here's to Life*. The year 2005 will be better, I know. I toast the air and repeat her refrain. "Yes, here's to life."

Chapter 9

The oncologists soon cried, "We found one, we have one! A clinical trial called Interferon and Bay 43, sponsored by Bayer Aspirin." That night in bed, as Bob lay sleeping, I placed my hand on his back and breathed a healing white light into his cancer, like a beacon of wellness returning again and again with each brightly lighted breath to blind the parasitic cells and banish them forever from his precious flesh.

Interferon had been used alone for cancer treatment but never in conjunction with an ingredient which the founders called Bay 43, whatever that was. Then began tests to qualify Bob for the trial. Cancer could not exist anywhere but in the kidney for this test. Bone scan, check. Chest CAT scan, check. Head MRI, check. Needle biopsy to legitimize his cancer for the paperwork, check. It's a go!

Bob, Judi, and I attended a cancer clinic session to learn how to inject the Interferon. But Bob took the lead in this, exhibiting the most determination of his entire treatment time. He administered all the shots himself—he who dreaded needles. (He was already bravely receiving massive injections of Botox in his neck for a condition called Dystonia.) Monday, Wednesday, and Friday were Interferon days and every day he ingested in pill form the new drug, Bay 43. We had great hopes. We established a morning routine for the Interferon injections. I was always a little nervous and probably so was he but never said so, and neither did I. Instead, we got through each session as Bob always got through life, and for which he was rightly admired: with a great positive attitude, with very well planned determination, and with humor.

At the clinic we had been given printed instructions which I continued to refer to at home. But, Bob, in his thorough and business-oriented fashion, transferred all the instructions to two index cards, which he filled on both sides. He numbered the steps and circled each number. There were twenty-seven steps and he took each one seriously and separately every Monday, Wednesday, and Friday morning.

He sat in the blue chair at the kitchen table; I, in the booth. Neatly, he laid out his cards and his injection materials: the aluminum tray with its clean lining, the Interferon "pen" as it was called, the needles, the alcohol and gauze, bandages, needle discard box. I unfolded my instructions and laid them out next to me. I was the moral support. No. 1 on the list was Wash Hands, which we both did. Referring to his list with every step, Bob persevered from taking the top off the pen to cleaning his leg with alcohol, checking the solution, inserting the needle in the pen, turning, filling, tapping, clicking in the designated dosage. Now we were at his No. 16, which was to roll and warm the pen in his hands, his strong, gentle, nearly shy, hands. I loved those hands. The actual injection was to follow this step, and that was the scary part, the climax in a way. By then I felt we needed some relief from our masked tension. In reality this was a poison we were putting into his body to kill his cells. In the guise of healing we were performing an act psychologically deep, dark, and sinister. I was always near tears.

Soon I knew the steps well. When he turned over his first index card No. 16 was next: "Roll capped pen in hands one minute to warm." Before he could turn the card I was doing the Interferon Rock and Roll. As the maraca-like pen passed over his wedding ring making music—click, click, click—I rocked my shoulders and arms to the rhythm. The injection today would go well, cha cha cha. No bent needle, no bruising, nor bleeding or pain. Cha, cha, cha. We are healing you, Bob, yah, yah, cha cha cha. Soon he knew when the Interferon Rock and Roll was coming, and as he turned the card over to begin No. 16 he would glance at me and smile. Of course I was smiling back—and dancing already. Click, click, yah, yah, cha, cha, cha.

Chapter 10

We began the New Year, 2005, with spiritual determination. My friend, Margie, sent me Science of the Mind Healing Treatments. I realized they were the Christian version of the affirmations and visualizations I do, mine being what I call with some flippancy, the pagan version. Actually, I was delighted to have this opportunity to discover yet another "connection," as all people and things connect in a metaphysical manner we are unable in our limited human form to comprehend. And we become less able to understand these connections as we continue sociologically and technologically to fracture ourselves into thinner more fragile and vulnerable shards.

I decided to adapt Margie's healings to suit myself. I would teach them to Bob. But how? I went to bed wondering what new magic I was conjuring up, what spells and protections I was reaching out for, what bit of ice covered stump I could grab sliding down, grasping onto Bob hard with my other hand.

Bob always believed in the power of positive thinking. "It's the greatest day of my entire life!" was his life-long mantra. Sometimes people were skeptical of his sincerity but his consistent repetition of this uplifting phrase eventually set a great example to everyone. He lived by it. So it was easy for him to incorporate another affirmation into the course of his life.

I suggested: "I am healing and I am becoming stronger." So after breakfast we did our stretching and breathing as usual. But before walking around the house, his morning exercise, he meditated on this phrase. I explained how people's minds wander in meditation and that he should just gently return to the affirmation. I reminded him to feel the words he is saying to himself.

He sat in the armless side chair in the living room, as he did each morning, the chair next to the small colorful table I bought in India. He sat straight; he remained quiet and calm, but not smiling. He had taken to wearing sweat pants at home and his slippers, though to the doctor's office he still wore slacks or grays, a belt on which I helped him locate a new hole, and Velcro sneakers. Less robust now, he had begun, for the first time in his life, to wear a light jacket outdoors. I sat in the armchair on the other side of the table. In retrospect, I envision myself fluttering around him like an anxious moth drawn to a steady, strong light. With his eyes closed, he was trying hard to concentrate and I was trying hard not to concentrate on him.

Now, in the present, after Bob has been dead two years, I think of my many meditations, or prayers as some would call them. Why couldn't I save him with them? Didn't I believe strongly enough that I could? Now I realize the meditations saved <u>me</u>. Through them, I protected myself, as well as Bob, from the demon composed of guilt, fear, doubt, resentment, and anger, like holding a cross to a vampire. You won't suck our blood, I hissed. You'll never get to me or past me to him. You will not wedge your evil form between Bob and me. Nor will you diminish our determination to grow strong and large and all conquering together. Dark creature, I will never allow you to infiltrate as deadly fodder for a glutinous cancer.

My journal entries for those weeks consisted of amulets: meditations, prayers, affirmations, some neatly numbered, others scrawled with emotion, some barely legible, as in automatic writing, others bracketed for emphasis. There were some starred and many underlined for rereading. A few were tear stained.

1/17/05 - Oh, my god it just hit me—he may be getting a placebo! In which case I had better get prepared with another treatment system in place! Beverly, stop crying, cry only a short daily bit and then do what has to be done. You are capable!

1/18/05 - Stiff neck, crying, overwhelmed by what to do next for Bob

1/23/05 - 5:30 a.m. Bad morning. Took half a tranquiller. Must keep releasing fear. Know that I am capable of following through.

1/31/05 - This week I must:
    1. Find a book for Bob on cancer survivors.

2. With Bob see a dietician to regulate blood glucose levels to starve the cancer.
3. Possibly consider Immunotherapy.

2/1/05 - Meditation: I take care of myself first because I am the caregiver. And I must live the life of Beverly, not that of Bob.

2/4/05 - Meditation: I live in positive belief that Bob will improve. Improvement leads to remission. I live in peace with this.

2/7/05 - Judi took me to the emergency because I was so dizzy. I was frightened. It turned out to be nothing, but the result of my having to go alarmed Judi, depressed Bob, and scared me when I realized all the responsibility I now hold for myself as well as Bob. Vowed to take better care of myself by seeing a therapist.

2/14/05 - This morning rushing around doing many things, including getting breakfast on the table, and Bob just standing there. I felt bad snapping at him, angry. I yelled, please just talk to me and tell me how you are feeling. So we sat and talked. He said he's sorry he will never be able to do certain things now, like take the RV to Montana alone on a fishing trip, but he wasn't sad. (I am sad for him.) I think we will be able to talk more now.

2/28/05 - 8:00 a.m. A new week, Week seven. Seven weeks of the Interferon Rock and Roll. Today we see Bob's oncologist to learn the results of the first CAT scan since he began the clinical trial on January 3. It will show if the cancer is shrinking or stopped. Sunny after so much rain. Feeling optimistic. I suppose Bob is as jittery as I am. I will awake him soon. What a bad dream our lives are just now.

The comparative tests for the Interferon and Bay 43 clinical trial showed that not only had the cancer not been contained, which was the hope for this treatment for there is no cure for kidney cancer, but it confirmed that the cancer had grown. We needed to find a different set of experimental drugs. Find another damn trial fast, I screamed in silence. Only now do I acknowledge this bravado and anger to be sheer panic. I can only imagine how Bob felt. He never said.

Chapter 11

I was nervous the first time I went alone to our mountain cottage on October 17, 2005, three months after Bob's death. Would I be able to face our tiny retreat where we had "played house" once a month for fourteen years, just he and I and our beloved black Lab, Oz? Upon arriving each time we would unpack in half an hour. "A turnkey operation," Bob always beamed, settling onto the cozy front porch facing the river, town, and mountains beyond. There is room for just two chairs there, brown, with a round table between for drinks and a wooden owl with one chipped ear we bought at the town fair one year from a man who spread his wares on the blanketed grass.

We would sink down with contended sighs and speculate on our chances of a perfect sunset soon wide above the far mountains. And where would we hike this trip? For there was always a morning hike, an afternoon rest and read, with maybe Scrabble and popcorn later and a rented movie at night.

On that first trip alone Bob's presence was so strong he did not feel gone, and I was comforted. (Only on subsequent visits, when I finally accepted I would never see him in Portola again, even as his spirit hovered, could I not stop crying. Once, in my walk in the hills, I ordered him to please take his dog and go to his boat! "Your spirit overwhelms me with loneliness today." So he released me to myself and I could stop thinking of him and stop crying.)

The only way to get through that first visit, I decided, was to remain in present time. I protected myself on all sides with a brick wall against fears and sadness. I could not have handled a melt-down. Nevertheless, Bob lingered close to my emotional boundaries. It was imperative I close myself to memories of happy times. I did not open the Portola picture album.

Instead, I concentrated on physical things needing attention, like overgrown trees, replacement of a water valve, new chores to learn.

I can handle everything, I told myself to feel confident and capable. This wonderful cottage is all mine now. Oh, Beverly, remove that sharp stab of guilt this selfish thought inflicts.

In October of 2004, exactly one year before my first trip back to Portola and weeks before the first blood clot, unbeknownst to Bob and I we were together there at our cherished cottage for the last time. But at the time, we were marking that visit in another way. Oz, our black Lab of fourteen years, had died. Sitting heavy and stony-faced on our hill beside the cottage we imagined him being in one of his many empty, quiet holes he had dug for his cooling comfort. That October, 2004 trip marked the first time we had returned since Oz died two months prior in August.

First time without Oz, last time together.

I knew there would be a full moon on October 17, 2005. But it did not find me until four o'clock in the dark early morning. "Awake!" Her glow echoed throughout my bedroom. I positioned myself in bed to stare out the window at her. I felt a cozy peace of mind that surprised me and soon turned to ecstasy. Is this how Bob felt when he said sometimes, "I'm feeling euphoric this evening"? After all, his astrological sign, Cancer, made him a moon baby. Now I knew why pagans danced in the forest in a circle of the moon's empowering light. I recited aloud: "The full moon gives me the power to hold and cherish the ecstasy of minute-to-minute life." As my body breathed in and out deeply, I thanked the moon goddess, my guardian angel, and my Bob for the peace I felt.

But I had to get closer. So, soon, out on the porch in twenty degrees and darkness, I was hunkering down in long johns, red flannel nightgown, robe, vest, down jacket, heavy sox, slippers, hat, and gloves. I watched the glorious moon set in the west. As the sky lightened in the east and the wispy clouds turned red I repeated the full moon power mantra: "The full moon gives me the power to hold and cherish the ecstasy of minute-to-minute life." On the last word, "life," the faint moon, so slight then I had to glance to the side to see it, disappeared behind the mountain. All around me the sky was a brilliant red. "See you tomorrow, Full Moon." But she hadn't really left me, for instead of setting into the mountain she had set into me. And we—Moon, Red Sky, Beverly—had melded into one. Into the magnificent, full, glorious past, present, and future.

Chapter 12

The roadmap from Catholicism to Moon Goddess covered years of miles. But regardless of its route, my long spiritual journey has influenced my grieving process, just as more conventional religion has helped many other widows and widowers.

The journey started for me when Katie, my father's cousin, took me under her Catholic wing. At seven years of age I was baptized and she became my godmother, after which I began the serious and frightening process of Catechism. Every Saturday morning in 1942 I ventured down, down into the dungeon-like basement of my first church, St. Elizabeth's in San Francisco. I sat on a folding chair near the back in the chilly hall and awaited the stern-faced nun whose name I have forgotten. Of course she wore the mysterious black habit, which in retrospective memory, now reminds me of a chador, that foreboding dark dress of some Muslim women. I was glad other children slowly filled in the space between my chair and the standing Sister.

The drilling of the lesson would begin soon and continue until we reached the highlight of the morning, the affixing of a colorful religious stamp into my gray Catechism book. The book contained rote question and answer chapters and prayers. I memorized hard all week for one of those pretty, large, square-shaped stamps of a saint, or God, or, if I was lucky, the Hail Mary. This reward was not like the tiny stars I got at school or from old Miss Glover at my piano lesson at her house, to which I walked on Tuesdays after school. There, I was stationed on a padded piano bench in her prissy front room, while she sat on an adjoining side chair with the small floor heater positioned to blow under her dress. Every week she placed a small star on the appropriate page of my book, but it was puny and always the same.

First though, the Sister at Catechism pulled down a rolled picture on a stand, like a map at school. Besides fearing the nun, this was the real reason I sat in the back. The picture she unrolled was not bland, with gently colored green and blue continents and oceans. This one showed, instead, dozens, or hundreds it seemed, of tiny red and orange evil, distorted creatures in various positions, some upside down, falling, all grimacing and suffering in cave-like surroundings full of fire, sinful lost souls writhing in Hell. Wide-eyed I could not look away, and I knew that would happen to me if I were bad.

So I stayed good and studied my Catechism. At age thirteen I was confirmed and took the name of Josephine because I was born on March 19, St. Joseph's Day. (Recently, my daughter, Judi, said she had brought the St. Joseph's metal to Bob in the hospital because Joseph is the saint of fathers. I did not know this.) Through my teens, every Sunday I walked the mile to Mass alone. (Years later I discovered the artist, Hieronymous Bosch, and there they were, all my little devils.)

As the years passed, that straight mile to church turned into a series of swirls, like those in poster art from the psychedelic sixties. The new map offered roads to the East: to yoga, reincarnation, meditation, questions; to the powers and possibilities of the mind; to the expansion of concepts, the inclusion of new thought, the revision of ideas, and the suspension of disbelief. For me, universes opened, magic was an option, and energy changed form but never dissipated or stopped traveling.

What a trip I made. In the end it seemed I knew everything and nothing. As a human being I was an evolving creature wedged between animal instinct and metaphysical mindfulness. The human brain can function to its limited capacity only. We humans can never know anything for sure. Like it or not, ironically, our amazing brains restrict us. About death, we each believe that which suits us, and that is just fine. It is more than just fine. It is the map by which we all contribute to the pattern of existence by connecting the dots to see the big picture. All roads on this map lead to the same destination. But our earthly intelligence, with its restrictions and limitations, cannot know the next step, the one after the death stop. So we trust that everything is possible; we believe that miracles occur.

Years ago I had my favorite dream. I was with others on a San Francisco street, all walking, going somewhere or nowhere, a crowded street, a vague feeling of knowing and yet not knowing everyone, a comfortable feeling. And then we scattered. Slender strands between us stretched and snapped free. Many people got on a bus then, but not I. (Just a month ago in another dream Bob boarded a bus without me and apologized for forgetting to remind me it was time.) In my favorite dream I had not missed the bus, but was destined to take an alternative route using a different vehicle.

At once, a bike appeared at my side. Feeling at peace and light-spirited, I waved as the bus pulled away. "I will see you at the end," I called. As I proceeded to ride my bike down a hill I noticed the wheels were not regular bicycle tires. Instead, I rested upon a body of sculptured, shiny chrome in the shape of an infinity sign, which is the swirl of an "S" on its side that connects to itself and returns. I rode fast with glee and was the first to arrive.

In the final scene of the dream I was standing in a dwelling that I knew to be a place of final knowledge. My arms were wildly open and outstretched to encompass all space. Smiling and joyful, I received everyone from their various travels into my open heart and absolute love, in a manner which in dream language I knew to mean: Finally we know the answer, don't we; we know ourselves, we have ourselves; we all chose a different way but we knew the truth would be the same, no more doubt, no more fear; we've been through it all, we have infinite wisdom; we have reached nirvana.

The sentence I uttered was short and commonplace, but it ecstatically meant all that. Standing there with my arms wide open I greeted them simply by saying, "Welcome to Bev's place!"

So, if we know that everything is possible in this life, then how do we live, I asked myself long ago. And now I ask, and how do I grieve? Perhaps the answer to both questions is the same. I believe the answer is that we must live fully in the present in our physical bodies in this physical world. Never mind that we have a memory of our immediate past and a penchant for planning the future. Never mind, too, that scientists and metaphysicians show us that objects are but fluid molecules vibrating at various rates of speed to appear solid. (Even still, we do touch rosy cheeks and smooth glass, crunchy snow, slick silk. I <u>know</u> I held fifty years worth of Bob's firm, protective, gentle hand in mine.)

Of course, some of us have developed greater spiritual capacities for transcendence from the physical world, but most of us have not. Nor should we necessarily do so and abandon our work here on earth. We are each an energy force of free will which has chosen the human form to be our guide in this plane. Therefore, we must nurture and protect that form and receive its wisdom. Our body's job is to teach us how to live. When our spirit, which is the essence of us each, has practiced the lessons sufficiently, or when it has completed its purpose here, it moves on.

Bob's soul moved out, and like his bodily house, I, too, was deserted. Of course I felt vulnerable, more so because I know we are born alone and die alone. And now I was alone. But he had to leave because his work here was done. I truly believe that, and furthermore, what is left, is for me to complete mine.

Chapter 13

The second clinical trial consisted of pills, but no shots, with accompanying meds for the nausea the treatment caused. Tuesday was pill day. After breakfast Bob would lift the tiny lids of the pillbox and begin the complex process of filling each of the seven compartments with that day's prescribed dosage.

"Oh, gee," I heard him mumble one Tuesday while he was doing the Jumble puzzle and counting out his meds. I turned to see he had mixed the days. The pills were so alike in size and color it would take some effort to sort them out properly. And the little squares rendered a tight-squeeze for any size fingers.

"Oh, honey," I complained and dumped them all out. "Let me do it." I stood over him identifying, resorting, and fuming. "Now which day are the blue ones?" In his humiliation he was quiet and still.

"Pay attention when you do these," I shot as I finished up. I never remember that incident now without shedding tears of shame and sorrow at my behavior that Tuesday. I remember thinking I must reduce my caffeine intake which was making me jumpy and emphasizing the difference between my frantic pace those days and Bob's unavoidably slower one. A champion Jumble player before, now he couldn't get the words, I noticed, and I pretended I couldn't either each day as I moved about the kitchen tidying up. He was anemic; he was foggy; and he was weak. How much to expect of him now, I wondered. How much of him to protect.

Then, one morning upon rising, he fell into his nightstand. That surprised us both. He did not go all the way to the floor and I was able to help him upright himself.

"I'm okay, I'm okay," he said, continuing on to the bathroom.

"You sure? I'll just wait until you're ready to come to breakfast."

But the second time he went all the way down in the living room. This was a totally strong, physically muscular man whose firm handshake often provoked comments and painful grimaces.

"Let's not panic," he said calmly from his position on the carpet. Thin, weak, and as a terrycloth-robed figure on the floor, he was, nevertheless, in charge. We both knew I could not lift him. But we had worked well together for fifty years and Bob had never panicked in any situation.

"Get the chair," he said.

"Yeah, that'll work." I turned the sturdy, straight-backed chair towards him.

"Now, I'll pull up and you take under my arm at the same time," he continued. We worked slowly.

"Ready?" he asked. One heave took him up. He rested in the chair and then continued into the kitchen.

But once, on a different day at lunchtime, he choked on water and the look on his frightened face terrified me. I thought he would die right there with me trying to give him a seated Heimlich procedure because that is all I could think of to do. "Oh, my dear Bob," I cried holding him in my arms on the booth seat when the water had cleared. We remained there quiet for a few minutes.

One early evening after Bob had retired and I rested on the couch, a new guide popped into my consciousness. Dwarflike and feisty, "You don't need Tunis now," he growled. I knew he represented the foursquare, solid, practical part of myself. "You need me to remind you to prepare not for dying, but for living," he continued. "When Bob teaches you how to do the chores and business of the household he is responsible for, do not be sad because he must give them up. Instead, consider them new skills you are adding to your repertoire of knowledge and experience." Poof, that was it. Didn't even leave his name. No nonsense. Just get on with it.

In time Bob could not rise from his chair. We got a walker, then a wheelchair. These are the challenges we were required to face now, I pondered one morning as I gazed at a red sunrise. But it came to me that there were other important challenges besides the physical ones. It was just as difficult a task to be challenged with accepting the joy as well. Suddenly, it seemed imperative I glean bits of these joys, the gold treasure of life, like this sunrise, and continue to present them with confidence and love to my dear Bob.

When we saw Bob's oncologist that month she noticed him stumble and ordered a MRI of his brain. She suspects brain cancer, I was thinking. I was sure it was the anemia and pills. She proved to be wrong. Then she ordered a bone marrow test because there was high calcium in his lab work. That was cleared also. Again I thought, she is determined to locate cancer throughout his body; that's her job. I, on the other hand, was determined to get Bob to Stanford for another opinion before the April deadline that would show if the second clinical trial had worked. Within that time frame I would try Chinese medicine, too.

March 19, 2005, arrived, and I turned seventy. As "Feisty" had counseled, I would just get on with it. The birthday motto for my next decade would be *see the humor in everything; take nothing in life too seriously; keep seeing the positive.* I invited our six oldest friends for lunch. Bob was refusing to see people, but I wanted him to be with his friends so he consented to the celebration. I shielded us both from the unacknowledged truth, that this would be the last time these old friends would see Bob. He probably knew it, too. Nevertheless, he wanted to make my birthday special, so with Judi's help he orchestrated surprises for me. He had a special cake made, with a dancing woman in an orange gown on it. Flowers arrived at the door. Finally, he arranged for one item to be delivered last.

"What does he mean he has something else to bring in? Where is he going?" I asked after the delivery person had rung, left gifts, and returned to his vehicle. Bob was sitting quietly with a view of the front door. He had that 'all will be revealed' look on his face, the look that I believe always signaled inner mirth for him. He had forever delighted in surprising me for my birthday. Once, in recent years, refusing to say where we were going, he drove us to an elegant, seven-course dinner at a gourmet cooking school restaurant. For another surprise he took me whale watching, even though he gets seasick on the ocean and indeed got desperately ill that time.

"What is going on?" I laughed. No one else knew either, it seemed. It was exciting. Immediately, the boy returned to our front door with two gigantic bouquets of seventy helium balloons, all colors. Judi and he squeezed them through the opening—they scarcely fit—and into the living room. Bob remained sitting in his usual calm manner, but he was smiling at his absolutely marvelous surprise. Soon we untied the long strings, releasing the big bubbles of color to fill the room as they bumped and glided drunkenly across the ceiling, healingly providing for us an aura of giddiness and laughter in which we moved through champagne and cake, presents and pictures, in merriment laced with anxiety. It was magical though darkly sad.

Chapter 14

It is ironic that Bob and I were independent individuals all our lives and yet neither of us had lived alone. (Another irony is that our lives paralleled each other's, from childhood in the same San Francisco neighborhood unbeknownst to the other, to our families' moves to Daly City, where we met at fifteen and sixteen in high school and stayed inseparable for the rest of our lives.)

But now, in this eighth decade of my life, I face living alone for the first time. Other grievers say, at least my husband has been spared this loneliness. That is the positive aspect of Bob's having never known the independence of living alone. Church-going folks claim we are burdened only with those hardships we can bear. Possibly that is a rationalization. But then, any belief system can be interpreted as such. Eastern religions say we are living our karma, or fate. Is this true?

I was the first child born to my parents, as was Bob. In those depression years, to have a job was gold. The work ethic was spawned as the innocent, honest, central entity of every family. It was necessarily revered and coddled. It thrived, as did the family, all the members of which sacrificed for the benefit of its growth. The adults worked long, hard hours, and by their absenteeism in the lives of their children, no matter how well intended it was, they passed on to their offspring the wisdom of work. In so doing, they inadvertently bestowed upon us the gift of independence.

For Bob, this independence channeled itself in various ways through the years and finally became distilled into the solitary, contemplative, peaceful activity of fishing, his life long love. I, on the other side of the yin/yang sign, turned outward, instead, to everything.

A 1963 photo shall remain forever in my mind as my passport to solo travel, another baby step to personal independence.

The figures in the photo are lined up in front of our opened front door, holding a butcher paper banner, and smiling: Judi, three, in her tutu and tights from dance class, Bob, in an around-the-house white tee shirt, Susie, (now Star), holding Swabie, our first family dog, a black cocker/dachshund mix. "Welcome Home, Mom" in colorful lettering stretched before them, as they held the sign up according to their heights. The charm of that crooked banner will always warm my heart.

I had returned from two weeks in Denver on my second Greyhound bus trip alone. (The year before, I had taken my first solo trip: a four-day Greyhound ride to Death Valley. Sounds like *The Life and Times and True Adventures of Beverly Kalinin, Pioneer*. In a way it was, for my grandmother in 1907 at the age of eighteen traveled alone on a train from St. Louis to a new life in the West. I believe we Americas have travel in our frontier blood, which I know I have passed down to my daughters. It was only a matter of time until it surfaced for me.)

I loved my Denver adventure: three days, two nights on a bus with people coming and going at various stations in the wee hours. At rest stops I would drag myself towards the florescent glow of the empty cafe, the idling bus behind me, its fumes thick in the warm, dark night. I ate stale pie and old coffee. I never skipped a rest stop; I hungered for all the experiences. Once I held a crying baby for a woman. We were all bus riders passing in the night. You asked where people were headed. I heard their stories about bussing. We were a kind of family, a community of people passing on through, some staying longer than others. Goodbye, good luck, we slipped from each other readily.

I was exhilarated when I reached Denver, and not completely because of the two-week writers' convention I would attend as one of the tuition winners. Actually, after the first week I became restless in one place. What I recall of the conference is not the lectures and classes but the day I played hooky to take a tour of Pikes Peak. And the time, like a wayward student, I slipped off campus, taking a few others, for pizza and beer.

Obviously, it was the venturing out, not the conference itself that fulfilled my longing for discovery. Returning home to that bannered welcome and seeing Bob I discovered something else: that I could depend upon him to sanction everything I needed to do in order to become.

What an emotional see saw! Independency makes us strong and sassy. Dependency is a weary warning that the human being is a vulnerable creature needing more than itself alone to stay balanced. In our fifty years married our dependence on one another kept us balanced. The brain and the brawn, we kidded; Bob physical and even-tempered, Bev emotional and high-strung. The man and the woman, the yin and the yang.

Now, with Bob gone, I work hard to stay sassy and brave because the dependency part scares me. There are no more welcoming banners for me to cocoon into and be safe. Alone, I maintain or change my house and its systems. Alone, I do twice the work physically, mentally, emotionally. I teach myself new skills and I make all the decisions. I assume sole monitoring of my health and energy. Alone, I watch myself trudge along. I hear warnings from friends. "Smell the roses." I have always smelled the roses. And whenever I drink a glass of wine I stand in the kitchen where I have poured it, gaze out at the trees and sky, salute the day, and make a toast to Bob. Still, the weight on one end of the teeter-totter is heavier now. When I haven't laughed lately I notice I am on the ground end of it and I cannot push off because there is no hefty sassy and strong me on the seat up high.

When I am on the ground I am mostly afraid. I have low energy, or I awake in the night with my mind whirling at a pace that prohibits my return to sleep. This anxiety links to worry, loneliness, restlessness, boredom, and bewilderment. And they all link to fear.

I have another picture of myself these days, another version of dependency versus independency. I am in my home taking strong control of business. I am surrounded by my lists, my writing, the chores, business calls, email, my television and books, my cat, the garden work, patio trees, pool serenity, and solitude. I have returned from being out there, maybe from a distant travel, perhaps just from local errands. Many widows cannot stand to stay in their homes without their spouses. For me, my home offers solace.

But there is more to this picture. My refuge is surrounded by a murky mote: fear. When I link across the bridge to the world and when I return to my sanctuary I am obliged to glance down into that mote. In the swirls and ripples of the opaque water I catch glimpses of loneliness. (I have no intimacy with another. No one loves me as Bob did.) I see concerns for my health. (That leg ache, that chest pain, am I well? Can I keep up physically?) Deeper still, where I cannot see beneath, I strongly sense the undercurrent of time passing. (What is my life now? What does my future hold? When will I die?) Every day I cross the abyss and I face fear. I hurry over the bridge and wrap myself up in the metaphorical welcome banner, which is my home. Or, I go out into the world where, as ironical as it seems, I know there is safely because there are people.

I have always considered myself a synthesizer, someone who brings together apparently disparate parts to form a whole, or at least make a connection to a whole. Life is like a jigsaw puzzle of a million pieces and when we fit some together it pleases us. Likewise, the bridge from my home to the outside provides me with a means of synthesis by which I connect to life beyond grief. Of course the fears still swirl about below. Can I handle everything alone? Should I move to a smaller place in another city? What would I do there? To what degree do I trust in and share with others? My mother's Alzheimer's Disease began at the time of my father's illness and death. Nevertheless, I continue back and forth across the bridge. It is my link; it aids me in my role of synthesizer.

I love roadmaps for the same reason: they link, synthesize, and connect. Maps bring me forward to future possibilities. When I plan a road trip I spread them on the floor and bear down with a magnifying glass. I study the routes across states, the magical symbols, the tiny mileage numbers between dots. Where colors vary I ponder the secrets of those spots. I pour myself further in. Ah, elevation, there will be mountains for the long look I love, the bird's eye view of life. Best of all I trace the roads, the paths of connection in black, red, and blue. The most difficult links to make are the very thin lines, like thread refusing a needle's eye. What will I see hidden there? From dot to connecting dot my vision will grow.

Bob and I moved into the suburban house I live in now, the one he died in, in 1968. We could have purchased one in the hills where it is quiet and unincorporated into our town. But hill homes are the suburbs of the suburbs. We decided on this one in the flatland, with its morning hum from two adjacent freeways and a train corridor. There are shops, businesses, and buses within walking distance. A major airport is up the road. Within a few steps we could head east, west, north, or south to anywhere in the world. I have never regretted our choice.

However, one day years ago I had a startling epiphany. What if Bob dies first, I thought; I will be alone in the suburbs! And now it has happened. Recently one morning I was struck by the quiet loneliness of the sunrise from my driveway and I remembered that revelation. Then something made me take two steps forward and turn my head just slightly. There, over the far house and through the trees near the deserted playground shone brightly, not the sun, but the top of the very red Riteaid sign a block away. I smiled. How silly, a simple "sign" from Riteaid reminding me: Okay, you can just cross through the park and onto the boulevard—there are people for you everywhere.

I flash back to a scene years before of Bob and I sitting pleasantly on our couch. Perhaps we sipped cocktails; maybe there was music. "Did I ever tell you I love dinner jazz?" Bob said many times, a kind of repetitious comment he loved making. "Yes," I would smile. Or, "No! Really? I didn't know that," I might tease. Oz, our beloved Lab who died the year before Bob and whose unexpected death Bob never finishing grieving, lay between us. What I have remembered all these years is that as we chatted Bob was stroking Oz's head and I was scratching his backside. I recall thinking then how sad it was that we were not touching each other instead. We allowed Oz in the middle to be our connection to one another. Over the years I have envisioned that scene and finally I have come to another response. Now I rejoice at the idea that Bob and I were so totally fused together by the link we both much loved, Oz, our synthesizer.

Chapter 15

A feeling I ignore lies just below my surface, sometimes still, sometimes rippling in demand of a response. I do not know what the feeling is called but I sense when it is likely to poke at me. Is that why I cross over my bridge to the world? To keep the feeling quiet? Sometimes it strikes with surprise force. I was attending a ceremony to honor a husband and wife for their devotion to church activities and to each other. Suddenly, I sobbed aloud and left quickly, embarrassed.

The feeling is not called fear. Fear lives in my mote; it's a predicable, cognitive entity. I know where it stays, and we negotiate. Maybe the feeling is named desperation. Someone once said that people live lives of quiet desperation. But that occasional tedium is the wallpaper of human existence, the dull ache everyone at one time acknowledges or ignores. On the other hand, a widow's desperation is aggressive. It finds the chink, it makes the stab. Or worse, one lands on the rack.

One Sunday evening, anxious and weepy, restless and confused, I tried to analyze my mood, which had come on gradually and peaked with intensity. I talked about it in my grief support group next morning. But I had no idea that in telling the story I would sink into a depth of emotion so unprotected that two members quickly hugged me and the leader called me the next day to make sure I was all right.

I had been to a small birthday party Sunday afternoon for Bob's mother who turned ninety-five. The group consisted of the usual people: Bob's two brothers and their wives and me. It was a pleasant, jolly lunch from the deli with chocolate eclairs instead of a cake. We laughed and made jokes about age. My mother-in-law, bright and smiling, wore a tiara my daughter Star had sent from Alaska, and I took pictures. We had fun. Star also sent a small picture album of herself and the girls, my granddaughters, showing events of the past year. Included was a picture of the greenhouse I had given Star for her 50th birthday, which I had not yet seen. Also, there was the cancer Wizard of Oz theme run in which they all participated (named in honor of Bob). The surprise party pictures from Star's 50th birthday were included. None of those special pictures had been sent me. My throat was tight as I looked at them.

We always play Poker after lunch. Millie told one of her sons to go to her bedroom for the carved poker chip rack made by her father, which she had given to Bob years ago. (Bob's grandfather, Abraham, is a man whose life my Judi has thoroughly researched in her quest for family history.) Four days after Bob's death, however, Millie had asked for the rack back from me to "keep in the family." Was my branch now removed from the tree? So I had wrapped it up for her 94th birthday the year before.

This time I did not feel like playing Poker. They got right into it with their usual energetic spirit, counting out chips from the coveted holder and playing a complicated variety of games. I sat back and watched a while and then left early while they were still playing. At home I felt fine until dusk when I could not shake the feeling of abandonment.

At support group, by the time I finished speaking I was sobbing. I remember I kept saying through my tears, "I work so hard alone. I keep working so hard. I am so alone and I keep working so hard!"

Then, too, there are evidences of tiny desperations, ones like secrets. Oh, I forgot I already took the laundry from the washer. Did I leave the living room light on all night? What in the world... how long have I been staring at the pattern of the placemat, my hand on the cup of cold coffee, my back bent and face low? I am gazing at a dawn sky but am compelled to rush into the house—something vague near those peaceful-looking clouds could envelop me. As if sleepwalking, I say aloud, "I'm so tired;" then I come to with, "what? I don't feel tired! What am I saying?" Sometimes I walk around the house whispering "my Bob, my Bob."

Closely aligned with desperation is pointlessness. Greek legend has it that Sisyphus spent the whole of his life pushing a huge rock up a hill every day, only to let it slide down and begin once again at the bottom the following day. While it may be true that we stay attached to this earth by our simple daily routines, the pointlessness of life for widows and widowers feels as heavy as Sisyphus' boulder. Musing about life's purpose comes to everyone occasionally and just as easily is released in attending to daily issues, like navigating a commuter freeway, planning a dinner menu, doing Christmas shopping, crying over spilled milk. Unfortunately, we mourners can't get past the spilled milk.

In grieving for Bob the pointlessness of life presses hard against my body. It stands toe to toe with me. We walk together; we dance together. I do the dance of pointlessness, but with style. Why have I not tripped, I wonder. The answer may be that I am fearful of losing control. Also, I know I am programmed to endure and survive.

Still, suicide is discussed readily in my support groups as a calm, logical, possible alternative. Some refrain from committing the act to spare their children, they say. Some have tried. Most of us, I suspect, are afraid to kill ourselves, whether with the help of pills or otherwise. We have become addicted to rationally balanced lives. None of us wants to go too high or too low. But then, I visualize the teeter-totter again. Ironically, that particular play equipment does not work when it is stuck in the middle. The pointlessness of this playground ride is to push off the earth and get up high. Why else each morning would I study the sky, look towards the treetops, and watch the birds fly by?

Chapter 16

Three months before Bob died I wrote in my journal, "Now the hard part begins. Bob cannot be left alone. I feel trapped, my wings closed and taped to my body." But of course it was Bob who was trapped. And I wanted my wings free to free him and to continue flying towards solutions for his recovery. Both of us were bound and struggling and I could not rescue him from the icy slope he must have sensed was just beyond our patio.

One quiet Sunday afternoon Bob and I were alone in our bedroom. Judi, who had been a constant help to me and guardian angel for her father, was away from the house. Star and our two granddaughters, Sienna and Terra, had not arrived from Alaska, as they would be doing within weeks for the summer visit and especially to be with Bob. At that time the house would become animated and active, charged with energy.

But now it was still, as we remained together on our respective beds, he in his hospital bed, me in the twin beside it on piled pillows to be at his level. We both gazed out through the sunny window wall into the patio where the olive, lemon, and lime trees, plus various perennial plants, grew. The Monstrosity, with its shelves of potted plants, some trailing long tendrils with decors stuck in the soil and small wind chimes attached here and there, stood against the brick chimney. I had found the eight by five-foot white wrought iron display shelf in the vacant lot behind the K Mart nursery. And Bob named it.

"We have got to get this." I burst in excited from my walk one Saturday morning. "They are throwing it away."

"Not me," Bob laughed after I had described the thing. He was eating his cereal. "We can't go pushing that through the neighborhood." Bob was a very private person.

"Well, I can," and off I went.

It was more difficult than I had anticipated. We live four blocks from K Mart and the weight and height of the object made maneuvering on curbs difficult. I had finally met my match in this found treasure. One time I found a small wheelbarrow. That was easy. Another time I was thrilled with the discovery of ninety-seven dumped primrose plants. I brought the car back for those. I do admit Bob helped me put into our truck a mangled rebar "sculpture" I named *Russian Winter* because it was shaped like a sled.

With the Monstrosity half way home I worried I might have a crash. This thing was nearly as big as a small car. Just as I began regretting my determination to bring it home I heard a man's voice from behind me.

"Need a hand, lady?" Being so intent on not tipping the shelf I had not noticed Bob back there.

"Oh you sweetheart," I cried, relieved. And that is when Bob christened it.

"God, what a Monstrosity!" And so on that Saturday morning a few years ago with the neighborhood free to watch the parade, with much chagrin, that very private, rather quiet, kind, helpful man guided me and the granddaddy of all my found objects all the way home.

Looking out the window that afternoon I thought about planting color spots and flower seeds there in the patio. I thought about Bob dying. Birth and death, living and dying, occupied my thoughts. Jarred up and down with alarming force and speed on the teeter totter those three months, I wonder how I made it. And now, though the ride is padded in slow motion and the pace reduced, I still wonder if I will be able to push off the ground each time. I glanced at Bob who seemed to be in a dreamingly reflective state that he usually avoided. Somehow, in that safe, private space, it seemed time for me to ask him an important question. I reached through the bed's railing to hold his hand and with both of us still gazing towards the patio, I asked, "Do you think you are going to die?"

"I don't think about it," Bob answered, so quickly that I knew he had. "I stay in denial. That's how I handle it."

I waited a moment. Nothing inside or outside moved.

"Then maybe we won't be able to say goodbye," I ventured.

"At the end, or at some time, it will be the right time," he answered, his tone as even as the air around us.

I felt as if we were making a movie and all the real life was out of camera range: the continuity girl in her torn jeans, the jumble of equipment cables, lights, extras milling and whispering, someone spilling coffee. I waited for the director to yell "cut." The hubbub would resume, wind would blow the patio plants and trees, and Bob would jump up. "Good scene," he'd say, with a peck of a kiss on my chapped lips.

As reassured as he always made me feel, this time I had not been completely soothed by his answer. "I wonder if I can wheel your chair into the patio so you can watch me plant marigolds," I said finally. But instead, we continued to lay there, heavy and immobile, staring out. As it turned out, later I did plant flowers for Bob to look at, but I never brought him out with me again.

Two months later, in June, at his routine appointment, the doctor ordered more blood and arranged for him to go directly into the hospital overnight. "It won't be long now," she told me privately in the hallway. As Bob and I waited together in the lab for the bed confirmation I thought of the doctor's remark. I had heard her correctly. I knew what the statement meant, but I had let it slide right down the hall with her and into the office. Instead, I focused my eyes and ears on the chemo nurse as she performed her duties, answered the phone that confirmed our bed, and wheeled us to the hospital and away from the doctor's evil remark.

The transfusion brought Bob's blood count up to ten, higher than it had been, which gave Bob a feeling of new energy. Lying in his own bed at home the next day he actually tried to exercise, lifting his thin legs, once so muscular and gorgeous. The juxtaposition in my mind of the doctor's remark to me and Bob's determination to get well broke my heart.

Chapter 17

Looking back, I see that during the first two months after Bob's death I functioned within a protective cocoon of my own making. I do not believe we should "keep busy", as people advise. Nevertheless, I was busy. First, there was the memorial, a beautiful and soothing event. I never missed a beat after that. With so much to do on my own now, it was a project in and of itself to decide how much I <u>could</u> do and how much to hire out. Could I maintain alone, I nervously wondered?

In the next months there was a fence contractor, a dry rot man, a house painter, a gardener. I discovered no one would service my plastic Doughboy pool. Bob had done it; I could do it. I labored with the cumbersome pool vacuum hose. Thank goodness for the filter/heater man. I picked his kindly brain. As he cleaned an overly dirty filter, I made voluminous notes. For the mountain cottage I enrolled in a monthly plumbing service and located a handyman for other jobs.

In a state of quiet panic I wound through the East Bay hills, an hour from my home, to the Delta where Bob kept his favorite possession, his beloved boat. To whom would I sell it? In a lot near my home our small RV needed attention. I went there regularly to start it up and drive it around, wondering all the while if I would ever take it out again. I owned so much stuff. In my whole life I had never lived alone, and now, at age seventy, I was responsible for so many things.

Then, there was the paperwork.

As I continued to challenge myself through those emotional, fear-driven days, I clung to a security blanket, my journal with its daily entries.

<u>July 15, 2005</u> (day after Bob's death)—Numb. Had Star and Judi call a few people. I sit upon a surface of Prozac-induced stillness as

thoughts and feelings run helter skelter just below. Dorothy pads in circles on the stripped hospital bed. Where is he?

July 16, 2005—First time alone in the house. I want to feel what it's like. At first slightly overwhelmed by so much house for one person. But that was my head thinking. The house is not empty. I feel not alone or lonely. It is just still. And that stillness is warm love all around me. I walked from room to room, it is everywhere. In our bedroom by the window I heard ticking. Both his watches are on my dresser, calling me. They've been there for days but I didn't hear them sooner. I'll wear the gold one I gave him for his birthday (June 29) even though he wasn't strong enough by then to push the button to light up the dial in the night, as he liked to do. The house has a fullness, it is not empty. When Bob was out of town, then it felt empty, different. Now I can even smile.

July 17, 2005—Our 50th wedding anniversary. Judi gave me fifty gold-colored roses from Bob. Star took pictures of me holding up our wedding pictures. Terra tried on my wedding dress and looked beautiful. She said she would like to wear it when she gets married. I am wearing my ring set and Bob's gold wedding ring all on one finger.

July 24, 2005—I am okay until I look at anything about Bob. I cannot go into his closet. It makes me feel headachy and tired. I keep the door closed.

July 25, 2005—I think of my own death by suicide and I don't know if I could ever do it. I read that possibly suicide victims cannot stand the idea of a future of fast and demoralizing decline into total dependency. Is that how Bob felt, that he had reached that point? Is that what he meant when, near the end, he said to Judi and me, "I'm telling both of you—this is not the way to do it!"

July 28, 2005—Two weeks. The mortuary man comes today with Bob's ashes. When he died he was wearing a Portal tee shirt and new dark green sweat pants Judi had given him for his birthday and no shoes. How was it for Bob, watching his body burn? The ashes were delivered in a plain brown plastic box in a heavy plastic bag. I removed the sack gingerly—ashes are heavy and dense. I held the bag, cried and walked around the house hugging the container to me. I talked to Bob. "We are in the kitchen and I sit you down in your place in the booth, while I sit in mine. I am so glad I have the house to myself today without anyone else here. Just you and me again. Later I will put you in your chair in your room, where you watched TV. It was an honor and privilege to have been connected so closely to you in this life for so many years of our lives. I love you. I learned to let go from you through your death, even though you could not let any physical thing go yourself. I am forced to let go of the most important thing—you. If I can do that, which I must, I can do <u>any</u> letting go. Perhaps that is why you went first—to teach me this as a guide to the next part of my life."

<u>August 1, 2005</u>—A dream: two buses, a crowd, separated from Bob. He didn't tell me which bus; he got on and left me behind. I felt angry, lost, but somehow vaguely I knew I would find the way. I was more hurt than anything because it seemed he didn't care enough to tell me which bus we (or I) should be taking. He tried to at the end, I saw him in the distance, but by then the crowd had separated us. Was it a crowd of angels?

<u>August 2, 2005</u>—So, is *grieving* about <u>acknowledgment</u>, then <u>hurt</u> and <u>anger</u>? What about <u>accepting</u> and <u>forgiving</u>?

<u>August 14, 2005</u>—One month today. Still numb. I limit my thinking of Bob to avoid those extreme sobbing sessions that I controlled for the nine months he was ill. In taking Star to the airport I talked a bit but got short of breath and headachy and had to stop.

Maybe the support group in September will help me release at a healthy rate.

<u>August 18, 2005</u>—I eat a lot, drink wine, watch television movies. It's okay. Bob will hang around and comfort me.

<u>August 20, 2005</u>—Physical grief: my heel problem, leg aching, sciatic nerve, off balance, feel heavy, so very tired.

<u>August 22, 2005</u>—Slept on Bob's side of the bed last night; felt as if I were lying within him, like a mummy, his body the secure and trusty wrapping on the outside. Was I?

<u>August 30, 2005</u>—Picked up prescription for my leg. When the pharmacist, a stranger to me, had finished guiding me through the new drug, he paused, looked me straight in the eye and said with deliberation, "slow down and rest." He was either an angel or Bob's proxy.

<u>September 14, 2005</u>—Two months. This morning I broke one of our Alaskan coffee cups and threw it away, but I don't remember which was Bob's and which one was mine. Which of us did I banish from the kitchen? I believe I always thought of those cups as one unit. Now half is gone.

Chapter 18

They say the holidays are the worst times for a mourner. For me, it is not the year-end holidays, but rather, to my surprise, it is my birthday which is most difficult to celebrate. Who will ever again care enough about me to deliver a seventy-balloon salute? (And when my mind drifts, I wonder this: if I live to celebrate one hundred birthdays will I look back objectively to Bob who died at seventy-two and think he was young enough to have been my son now?)

Instead of receiving balloons on my following birthday, the first one without him, I was surprised by Bob in another way. To begin with, for the first time ever, I had no thought of the approaching date until Judi came over one day.

"Hey, your birthday's next week," she reminded me as we folded laundry in the hallway where the washer and dryer are installed in a nook. As if she opened a closet I had nailed shut, memories of special gifts from Bob spilled out. I had placed the last one, a delicate pink hummingbird lamp, on my jewelry stand at the entrance to my bedroom. I glanced at it over the sheet I was working on. When I went out at night I always lit it, a beacon from Bob for my safe return.

"I still have the first birthday gift Dad gave me when I was only fifteen," I said suddenly. "That's amazing, isn't it?" Judi smiled and continued folding with precision, even panties, which I never fold at all.

"It's somewhere buried in the garage," I said. Right then I decided to make a birthday shrine of some of his gifts. Abruptly I left Judi to finish up and rummaged in the garage. "...somewhere on a nail," I muttered, clearing cobwebs.

"Here it is!" An old wood-framed tennis racket, a classic. In what year had we last played? In the 70s? The 80s? I propped it up on the jewelry stand, where it scarcely fit, and hurried about for the other items I had saved. Now I was on a mission and I think Judi was entertained as she continued to fold and watch.

There. The gold stretch bracelet engraved "Love, Bob 12-25-52." Well, that was only three months from my birthday. It counts. I put it near the lamp.

"Remember this?" I asked Bob's picture on the wall by my bed, as I placed an oak music box next to the bracelet.

In 1954, before we had been married, Bob and I saw a stage production of South Pacific. The music box, which was my birthday gift that year, played two tunes from the show: "Some Enchanted Evening" and "I'm in Love with a Wonderful Guy." All these years the box has functioned perfectly. I wound it up and we listened to the tingling melodies until it wound down and stopped. Then Judi sauntered back to the laundry and I remained sitting on the bed between Bob's picture and the music box.

Now, in over fifty years that music box has <u>never</u> misplaced, or skipped, or shown any other signs of malfunction. It started promptly when wound up and stopped only when it ran out, with the tunes slowing at the end, or when someone deliberately turned it off with the little knob. It worked perfectly and with reliance. But that day, near my birthday, with Bob looking over my shoulder, *that special music box turned on and off all by itself.* It began, played one song only, *I'm in Love with a Wonderful Guy,* and then stopped.

I sat frozen as it started to play, aware that someone or something was in sync with me completely. Judi slowly reappeared in the doorway. Without speaking, we both stared at the playing music box. And when that song ended, the music box turned itself off. We waited a bit, still without talking, but the second song did not begin. Finally, with a twinkle in her quiet voice, Judi said, "How about the other one, Dad?" We grinned at each other, but Bob was only giving me that one special song. Soon, Judi returned down the hall, but I remained sitting in the warm silence, basking in the aura of a glowing room. I was in no hurry to leave that fine feeling.

I read somewhere after that incident that the easiest way for a spirit to communicate with us is through the medium of sound. I loved hearing that, needless to say. So when I was given another "hello" from Bob later, I quite cheerfully accepted the greeting as if he were in the kitchen with me, having a beer.

Bob had loved The Three Stooges, those head-banging, eye-poking comedian clowns. He watched them for hours, laughing uproariously. So, his dear friend, Leo, gave him a bottle opener with a picture of The Three Stooges on it. When a bottle was opened they recited a litany of one-liners. "How 'bout a beer? Coitainly! Yuck, yuck." (Pouring sound) "Arf, arf, arf, yeowllll!" When I have a beer, of course I use the opener. I listen, smile, and set the opener down on the counter. "Here's to you, Honey." I always raise the bottle and gaze out the window for a minute before moving on.

One particularly warm day, when I had decided to have a beer break by the pool, I went through the kitchen bottle-opening routine. "How 'bout a beer?", etc. I lay the opener down on the counter near me, as always, and raised the Sierra Nevada towards the window. "Here's to the day and to you, Bob." The sun shone brightly that afternoon, with no wind ruffling the trees. There was no movement outside the house or in the kitchen. And then, through the stillness, the beer opener, which lay perhaps eight inches from me on the countertop and which I had not again touched, began its message and repeated it all the way through. "How 'bout a beer? Coitainly! Yuck, yuck." (Pouring sound) "Arf, arf, arf, yeowl!" When it had finished I waited, without moving. In a moment I sensed the communication from his side had ended. I felt peaceful. I said out loud, simply, "Thanks, Bob, I miss you." The kitchen felt different to me as I crossed the floor, as if everything were standing still except me. What was happening? Had Bob's spirit actually been here, I wondered? And if so, was it still near by? And I was walking away from him?

Chapter 19

As enjoyable as holidays can be, they exist always as a transitional intrusion upon our daily routines. And we whose spouses have died are in transition already. So, as holidays come around we are forced to deal with not one but two transitional upsets.

In the first transition, the holiday one, celebrated in general by most people, routine life is put on hold in December. People shop, wrap, party, decorate, eat sweets, drink eggnog, laugh at gatherings, smile at children, and twinkle back at all the lights. "See you after the first," means "don't bother me with life now, I'm celebrating, I'm vacating."

The second transition, the grieving one, needs no description. We widows and widowers are simply struggling to get from there to here, from then to now.

Now, if we overlay one transition upon the other, like a transparency, we will see a graph of conflicting and intersecting spikes and dips representing events, emotions, and anxieties as frantically and as challengingly packed upon one another as exhausted shoppers on Christmas Eve.

This picture presents an image of the painful holiday legacy of mourners.

On the first Thanksgiving without Bob I felt like a Pilgrim, a pioneer exploring new territory, as we drove the three-hour holiday freeway clogged with cars full of angst and family foreboding. Judi and I had invited ourselves to Bob's brother's house in Sacramento. We were starved, not for turkey but for stories of Bob and Thanksgivings past. In their chandeliered dining room, Dick and Darrene served the Kalinin dinner originated by Bob's mom. From the smoked salmon and pickled herring (which Bob disliked), through the relish-plated salad, complete with stuffed eggs (which Bob loved) to the fat turkey and traditional pies, the dinner table stayed well garnished with relatives and laughter. I devoured the garnish. Though my large van felt empty as Judi drove us through the dark back to home, I would say that the first of the big four had gone as smoothly as possible.

The holidays rake people into family piles, leaving only lines in the sand. Judi and I clung to each other on the long, dry stretch of empty beach. For Christmas Eve my friend, Louise, never missed a beat. "Come to my mom's house." Needy Judi, needy me. We allowed ourselves to be warmly enveloped by this generous clan. Two down and counting.

Star, in Alaska, had chosen to remain there for the winter holidays, with her new partner and, of course, her daughters, my granddaughters, Judi's nieces. But this Christmas I would not abandon Judi who could not leave her job. In November I had topped three small pine trees on my country property, two for my city patio dressed with colored lights and the third for a table in the living room. At night the tree lights twinkled their sham of former normalcy, even as they assuaged my pain. Nevertheless, every gift without Bob's name was a reminder. I spread out the sparse packages and avoided reading the tags.

One year Bob had decided I should have an abundance of presents to open to match the stacks of gifts I provided our girls. So he purchased many small items.

"Oh, you got me so many," I remember whispering to him on Christmas morning, glancing over my presents to the others' generous piles, fearing they may not have remained larger than mine that year. He had purchased lotions, jewelry, soaps, sox, and so much more, and wrapped them as he always did with wrinkled paper, crooked tape, and mismatched bows. They were priceless.

That first Christmas both Judi and Star came through with their own versions of Bob's precious packages. Judi made sure I had many small gifts to open. And Star sent gifts for Judi, Dorothy, the cat, and me from each member of her human and animal family, of which there are four people, four dogs, three cats, two gerbils, and numerous fish.

On Christmas morning Judi and I drank strong coffee and nibbled chocolates as we opened our gifts and filled the vacuum with scattered wrappings.

"Here, put Dorothy in the middle of her creams," Judi ordered as she took pictures of us. I had bought and wrapped a carton of the little restaurant creams to which my cat seems addicted.

"If I can get her out of the catnip," I laughed. The caffeine and candy fueled our efforts to be jolly.

Later, dressed in our holiday best, for our Christmas dinner I took Judi away from my empty dining room for a Christmas dinner at the elegant Equinox Room on the top floor of San Francisco's Marriott Hotel. Though we were afforded all views of the City by a slow evolution of the restaurant, I felt it was we who were centered and stationary, with the City moving to hold and support us, whereby providing profound grounding and peacefulness. And each time we faced west, the sun had set a degree more on our first lonely Christmas without Bob.

Chapter 20

In the ancient Tarot cards there is one called the Fool, a carefree figure pictured on the cliff's edge. Against a yellow background he wears a short, outlandish orange and brown dress with wide, flowing sleeves, the kind of outfit I would like. His hair is longer than mine; he could be a woman. There is a knapsack dangling from the stick over her shoulder and a tiny white flower in her other hand held high. A small dog romps at her heels. The Fool's face is tipped to the sun. As a free spirit he celebrates spontaneity. It is hard for me to accept the fact that this adventurer cautions us to be aware of dangers inherent in testing our limits. But that is exactly what he does.

I am heartily drawn to the Fool.

For the fourth holiday I dreaded meeting the challenge of the new year's symbolism. Bob had liked to celebrate New Year's Eve with steak and champagne at home and go to bed early. Now alone, that would not work for me. Instead, I decided to do a New Year's Eve ritual based on the Fool spell box my friend, Susan, had given me for my birthday that year.

Along with a small matchbox that came in a rich, gold-tasseled burgundy bag there was a tiny harlequin mask smiling guardedly from beneath his three-pointed, tri-colored cap. Also, there was a white candle adorned with the Fool's picture. The matchbox contained tiny images and symbols to help me focus on my present and future life. The Fool's picture on the box as well represented the theme for me: a free spirit moving forward with caution.

On the eve of the New Year 2006, when it was dark outside but hours from the traditional countdown in New York, I sat comfortably upon a straight-backed chair with my feet placed flat on the carpet. I had chosen this spot in my living room because in it I felt both centered (I did meditation there) and open (I could see much space in two rooms around me.) I placed all the items on the side table where

I kept small sacred symbols given me over the years, like the statue of Quan Yin, Goddess of compassion.

First, I lit the candle. Then, from the box I removed the little metal chalice, representing "Cups," a suit of the card deck which stands for our capacity to feel, dream, and imagine. I said aloud, "I assign this symbol the heavy chore of helping me sort and temper my feelings of sadness and loneliness. I beseech help in imagining my future and dreaming it into some kind of peaceful reality."

Next to the chalice I set the one-inch sword, reminiscent of the one on my girlhood charm bracelet to which always I felt alienated by its connotation of violence. The suit of "Swords" makes me feel the same. But in the Tarot the sword signifies our ability to be thoughtful and analytical. If this weapon can function as a tool for cutting away my angst and for trimming my thoughts and worries into sharp manageable pieces I would gladly assimilate the sword into my ritual.

"I am placing you precisely," I continued, then patted it lovingly to temper its might. "Please allow me concise thinking in planning a life without Bob," I said.

"Pentacles" symbolize the need of humans to feel our innate connection to nature and to our physical selves. I lifted the star in its circle, turning it round and round in my fingers. Circles are soothing to me because of their relation to nature. At once I visualized a green tree. I felt myself relaxing, melting down, drawn into my body which guides me in this physical world and then into the earth through my feet on the floor. Down, like roots flowing through the ground to the earth's center of molten heat from which I draw energy to live well.

I placed the little pentacle with the other charms and sat quietly feeling my connection to all life. I was on the edge of what I call ecstasy, but, as always, that divine state alluded me. Instead, I accept that to feel joy is to know the height of my bliss on this side of death.

Finally, the fourth suit is represented by a wooden match, which is "Wands," signifying the desire to create and ability to take action. As I examined the match I saw a torch held high. "Such bravery," I murmured. I imagined the flame. Tears came to my eyes for the courage of all human beings, all of us struggling. Then I felt the steel shaft of the torch supporting my straight spine. I saw the fire bursting from my crown, the earth's hot energy fueling me, the bright wand lighting the path ahead.

I lay the match near the harlequin mask. His smile caught my eye and I smiled back, taking this as a sign to draw on his sense of humor in the new year of 2006, the year in which Bob will not laugh with me, the first full year of many without him.

I moved in my chair and sighed. There were three other symbols to consider—a packet of herbs, a stone bead and a miniature Two of Pentacles card. I did not know what herbs are contained in the tiny, shiny silver bundle but I trusted their power nevertheless. The stone bead is purple amber, and I did know it is the highest spiritual color in the human aura, which is the energy glow that emanates from our bodies. I revere all stones and rocks regardless of color for they are small samples of our Mother Earth.

I found I related to the serious Two of Pentacles without hesitation. How happy I was to discover from a Tarot expert that he is cousin to Fool, for he holds in his arms a miniature eternity sign which looks just like the bicycle in my favorite dream, the one I rode a long way to Bev's Place to reunite with all my friends at journey's end. But he <u>does</u> represent such a lot of heavy work in this life. I long for him to release the burden of the infinity sign and, instead, climb on and ride and glide easily, as I did in my dream. The bright yellow Fool, light with flamboyancy, appeals to me more, even as he cautions me about dangers. Nevertheless, I will concede to his cousin and carry my prescribed portion of infinity—in between the times I hope to be dancing on the cliff.

Chapter 21

It seems I consider myself a free spirit and an adventurer, but the jolt I suffer from having turned off the main road is debilitating. The scenery of this new direction along the cliff, though to others may appear familiar, casts for me a different shadow. The light slants from an unexplored angle. Dancing there I believe myself to be the same person as I have been forever. I am what I am, I assure myself, but what is that? Without the mirroring affect of my partner, who will define me?

Since Bob died I have had the unsolicited opportunity, indeed the urgent need, to reexamine my relationships with everyone. On this road I see people in the new light. I look for my reflection in their mirroring profiles.

First, I see an independent, unconventional in-law who did a great job caring for a sick member of the clan. She had been strong and persevering. Even as she is alone now she will do fine. She had been married to one of the most well loved members of our family in all his roles: son, brother, brother-in-law, cousin, uncle, grandfather, father. Finally, I see the perpetual big sister, always stable and responsible, married to a favorite brother-in-law.

As for my daughters, I see myself in an image of life-long mate to their beloved father. I loved that our two daughters placed their father on a pedestal rightly deserved. It was easy for the girls mostly to prefer such a kind parent, an easy, non-confrontational man, a father supportive in every situation regardless of the circumstances, one capable of avoidance and passive aggressiveness, tactful in conversation and skillful at withdrawing when he found it necessary.

They adored their father, but of course they mourn him differently than I do. They have become bereft of fifty percent of their parent package. They cast a fleeting, worried glance at the other half, but she is strong and doing so well. They are proud of her. She will get along fine with time. Nevertheless, they wouldn't want to lose her, too, I read in glancing over at their profiles.

(<u>We</u> lost <u>them</u>, however, in their teens—even as they returned to us much later. Their leaving was not gentle. In the vernacular of that day, they split, each to her individual destination. There was no reassuring statement like, "I am off to college or to another adventure, but I will miss you both and I will return." Instead, their quick getaways carried the same message: you have served your purpose, goodbye, if I ever need you again I shall let you know.)

As for friends and others, the roads they travel are all inland. I wave at them; they wave back. Bits of reflection flash at me like fleeting mirrored sun catchers in the wind: We think of her. Quite a bit. A little bit. She's strong. She's lonely. She'll get through. We care. She does well. She's strong. She's alone.

No matter what I see in the various mirrors near and far the fact remains I am alone. After Bob's death professionals warned me that relationships with others might change. I did not understand how that could be true. I do not think I believed them. But if this premise is correct how will it manifest itself amongst the family now that my link to them, my spouse, is missing?

As widow or widower our previous life had been created by a series of persons and events attached on end through the years. Therefore, how can any of us regard family members in the same way we did before the death occurred. How can we possibly do so when our biggest role, that of spouse, is now nonexistent. That link is gone. We survivors are no longer husband or wife.

If I am not now "wife," I am a single person. Like the millions of other single people in the world, I have only myself. I need to learn to care for myself totally now because there is no longer another in my life to do so. And at this time of life I am all I can handle. With this major change my days of caring for another are at an end. Those names by which I have been known have not disappeared, but they have been diminished by my new status—names like mother, grandmother, sister, aunt, and in-law. They are labels that have faded. The strength of a chain intact no longer exists. The broken part hangs heavy, its icy bulk a burden. I want to let go. I need to <u>feel</u> free spirited again. That is how I have lived my life. That is how I choose to grieve.

As the weeks pass I allow myself brief, fragile glimpses into a possible future. Some widows and widowers seek other partners immediately (though it is mostly men who remarry.) Not I. Because I have functioned in an independent fashion most of my life, I embrace the fact of my alone self and will deal with the loneliness as I can. The future I glimpse may form two main alternatives: I continue exactly how I have lived but without Bob, or, I change directions completely.

Bob said I was brave. Whether speaking out against the majority or pushing his doctors for correct treatment, I want to remember I always have acted forcefully. Bob said I was a tiger. I liked that. He and I each took pride in being our own person first, a devoted mate to the other second. Can I be that independent person still?

Of course, changing directions for the future is the harder option, a frightening one. Where would I live? Whom would I meet? What would I do? But to refuse honoring my new existence, I may be dragging along forever that chain of old labels, the weight of which restrains my life in place. With a new layer of ice forming around each role each season, I will continually refreeze at zero degrees until there is no cracking out. "Oh, that bump is mom; that one over there, the grandmother." I will quietly freeze to death.

I love my daughters desperately. I love my granddaughters far away in Alaska. I long for them to know fearlessness and a joy in living. I want them all to be in my life always. I love family members and old friends; we have history together. But I am Beverly. I am alone. I am fiercely individual. I need to move on.

The relationships in our lives before our spouses died comprise what I call the "living past." For the most part, those people still are there, thank goodness. They have the same titles they had before: *son/daughter, sister/brother, niece/nephew, cherished friend*. But we survivors are no longer *husband* or *wife*. The broken chain represents our living past. In new positions, we without titles dangle free. We are scared, excited, and anxious, but resigned mostly to go forward, because now we are our own "living present."

So, Fool that I may be, I drag a heavy chain at the edge of a cliff. To maneuver with ease, do I dare remove it from my ankle? Is there any way I can hope to crack through my frozen state? Surely the powerful sun can melt any impediment to my dance.

Chapter 22

As I pass the second-year anniversary of Bob's death, I remind myself that the only cure for grief is grieving and that a new life may take years to reprogram. Do we have enough time left to reach a new "normal?" And yet we know that a deliberate, well-planned grieving period insures that we will not be having a breakdown later. We must not push our emotions either down or away, tucking them safely into the secret soft tissue of our vulnerable core or keeping them at a stiff upper arm distance from ourselves while we linger behind a brick wall.

But regardless of how essential it is that we take time to cry and allow sadness, nevertheless, memories hurt, <u>the good ones as much as the bad</u>. I visualize Bob laughing hard, his face crinkled, eyes closed, grabbing his chest and leaning back or forward into that fun, infectious place of overwhelming joy, surrender, and release. Everyone loved watching Bob laugh. For a moment I smile seeing him in my mind's eye. But soon my mind is distracted by a sensation of suffering upwelling from my center to my shoulders, neck, throat, face, a wave gushing out my eyes, stifling breathing, causing pain as it crashes into my skull, from which there is no more escape. After a while I allow breathing to return, which assuages the storm within my body. The wave recedes and, finally, I am becalmed.

Or, I remember Bob offering a hug, arms outstretched. He joked that I was like a little hamster needing handling every day to remain happy and tame. "You didn't have your hug today," I hear him kid, and I leave the kitchen sink or the dusting to be in the warm enclosure of his bear-like embrace. At this memory, again the storm rages within me, leaving me weak and broken at a time when I am just rebuilding.

So, why submit myself to these good memories? I do not know how much grieving I can take to cure myself. How much "healing" can I stand? It seems that in order to heal I must again consider the balancing act: how much must I recall of our fifty years together, and how much shall I allow to settle into my unconscious past, as have the lost memories of childhood. (I grew to a stable adult without recalling them.) Alzheimer's patients forget all and often remain happy in the moment. We are the sad ones for their memory loss because we are part of their past. My mother was quite merry being with me nearly every day, even as she had forgotten almost everyone and everything else.

I saw a movie recently, "Reign Over Me," in which the man had lost his wife, three children, and pet dog all in one accident. He self medicated by forgetting he had had a family; he went crazy. What is the precise degree of healthy balancing between remembering and letting go of remembering?

It has been two years, and I have not cleaned out Bob's closet yet. When will I? I hear the experts say, as we all have, that it takes everyone a different amount of time. The myth of one year is debunked, everyone knows who has lost a spouse. There is no miraculous return to "normal" because "normal" is dead. You do not get *over* your husband's death, the professionals say; you get *through* it. And you are different on the other side.

That sounds as if we have entered a rabbit hole, but contrary to Alice's experience, there is no cozy bunny home to rest in. There are cold, dark, scary, damp, dirty twists and turns we claw through in a claustrophobic sweat, with black earth pressing under our nails and our red scraped knees beginning to bleed. We fear most of all that there will be a dead end. And if there is not, what will await us on the surface should we make it through? I am beginning to suspect there will be space, only space. We will breathe and wipe our hands and faces. With effort we will hoist ourselves all the way out and sit on the green grass. When I look around at the infinite space, I am sure I will notice a teeter totter way over there, the one we all use, the one I will play on for the rest of my life.

I suspect that when I make it through I will feel exactly the same, only numbed a bit because the entry hole was years over in that past direction. How many memories will I have lost or released in the dark passageway? Would my journey have been easier without the burden of so many recollections? Perhaps there was a designated place for them in the tunnel. Along the way, will I have filed them under "living past?" Regardless of all these considerations, the primary question remains for me. And that is, in order to <u>heal in the best way possible</u>, should I deliberately allow more of the memories, good and bad, to slip away?

Chapter 23

Perhaps real healing does not commence until we are ready to replace the pain with forgetfulness. I first began thinking of this theory at Portola, in the mountain cottage Bob and I shared for years. I go there every month and each time the degree of sadness I feel differs, with no consistent pattern as to intensity. On some visits I am light hearted, on others I sob. I am trying to make the cottage my own.

On that particular early morning when I considered the benefit of discarding memories, I had just made coffee while glancing at the rosy sky. I was anticipating my dawn-time sit on the porch. The mountains were out, with one or two pink clouds near them. I felt wide open, like the sun that would soon provide bright possibilities for a new day. Rays of energy streaked from me in micro moments of forgetfulness that Bob had died. Of course I remembered immediately, but I wanted more of that absence of sadness. Were those brief slivers of joy healed splashes of my emotional self? How could I foster their increased number?

In watching for other incidents of healing that morning I noticed they occurred when I planned the day's hike, as well as when I studied a nearby bevy of quail with binoculars. At neither of those times was I recalling Bob at all. I had not thought, as I am prone to do, those were Bob's binoculars, or, Bob and I would be hiking in the Lakes Basin area this day. Those special recollections would not have provided healing, I sensed. Instead, I determined that instances of true healing—not just scabs covering festering wounds—would continue to occur when 1) I experienced short but complete periods of forgetting and 2) I was fixed in the absolute present moment in time. Furthermore, I would not have reached those healed moments that morning if I had not gone through the past two days of crying.

Suffering, as I did those two days, is part of the prescription for healing. I tell myself often that the only cure for grief is grieving.

Mostly, suffering takes the form of remembering. But what is the proper and adequate strength of this medication? I refuse to forget Bob, but I need to switch to the channel of the movie of my life now. I need to step away from things past.

Recently I attended the fortieth anniversary celebration of the Summer of Love in San Francisco's Golden Gate Park. The meadow of thousands undulated in tie-dye while familiar sixties scents wafted through the air. Hearing the hallucinatory-induced old music was like holding a security blanket. One could feel safe, loose, flowing, and free.

I had to park a half-mile away, but I did not care. It was a gorgeous day and the cozy dirt pathway to the meadow soothed me with both splotches of mottled sunlight and rich damp shadows from the greenery all around. "I am loving every step of this," I thought breathing in the moist aromas. "I am fully in the present." I would be revisiting history, but I knew I would not be recalling memories. I kept thinking, "On this day, at this moment, I have definitely switched to the channel of the *Movie of Me Now*."

By the time I had reached the meadow with its musty music and sweaty bodies I had become focused into a fully grounded emotional place as both a participant and an observer. "I am alone in the world now," I thought, "but I am surrounded by people. Bob was my rock. Now I am my own rock." I swayed to the music, I walked to several different spots through and around the crowd, and I looked into people's faces.

I did not need to stay long, and on the way back to the car I stopped at a lake, bought a hot dog, and watched a sailboat float back and forth. Where was the owner? I searched the rim of the water. And that is when the remote control took over. Suddenly, I was zapped back to a snapshot of Bob by a lake with our three-year old Susie, our first daughter, in her warm, blue, matching coat and hat shaped like a bonnet. With caution, she was feeding a squirrel a peanut. Bob, the strong guardian, in sport shirt and a light sweater, kneeled close to her, smiling, proud, and happy.

I had gone rapidly from the history channel at the Summer of Love anniversary to the channel of the *Movie of Me Now*, and then swiftly to the memory channel—a lake, the City, the ocean beyond.

Now, remembering my life with Bob, which was everything after I turned fifteen, was engulfing me.

Driving home I felt even sadder as the entire way resounded with memories of a life all gone. Along the beautiful Crystal Springs reservoir near San Mateo, I discovered I had reached some clarity between memory and history. To review history, as I had done at the Summer of Love festival, is to live in the present. It is an activity of current life and life is <u>not</u> sad. "Living," by its very definition, that we are conscious entities, must be considered as glorious. A lifetime of memories, on the other hand, packed to overflowing with Bob, who is dead, is devastating. <u>Therefore, in my mind, the trick is to convert memory to history.</u>

In the Mexican celebration of Day of the Dead there is a saying: We die three times—when our soul leaves our bodies, when we are buried, and when the last person living who remembers us dies. Bob will not be forgotten in my lifetime and for some generations following. But he is a part of my history now. So, let me recall him as history, which is a great component of life and, therefore, <u>not filled with sadness.</u>

Perhaps the hardest kind of memory to surrender is the nostalgia of past years we shared only with our dead partners. Roaming San Francisco's financial district recently I decided to search out 333 Montgomery Street where I was a nineteen-year-old stenographer. I always have loved the Kathryn Hepburn/Spencer Tracy movie, *Desk Set*, because it portrays the 50s office scene so well and reminds me of my first job—the white gloves and hat of the exciting big-city commute, the camaraderie of the "girls", the efficiency of and pride in our shorthand notes, the gossip, and the traditional Christmas party where at least one of the stenos got a little drunk.

Sometimes Bob, a U.C. student still, would meet me for lunch at a small sandwich shop in an alley off Pine Street around the corner. It was a date, as exciting as any could be, with my future husband. Maybe I would be wearing my favorite gray dress with the matching bolero jacket. Certainly I had on high heels, possibly the red patent leather ones Bob liked. (Four years later, when Bob had been hired by Proctor and Gamble and worked downtown himself, we met again for lunch, this time on Market Street, he in a new suit and tie, and I with his two-year-old daughter, Susie, who wore white gloves on the streetcar from our apartment on Eighteenth Street on upper Market.)

But 333 Montgomery Street as I had known it did not exist anymore. The building had been remodeled and redesigned. The old front entrance was no longer recognizable. Here were nostalgic memories that, without Bob to continue sharing them, had no value. I do not want to become melancholy thinking that no one but me knows those times now. If I could, would it not be better to banish them from my memories with a remark like, "they were precious, but everything changes always. They are history, and I am here now."?

The history channel and the channel of the *Movie of Me Now* remain side by side on the dial. Their positions require delicate manipulation to stay balanced, especially when the remote control wand, as if bewitched, slides me into memory. Then I end in tears. Why must I dwell there?

It is bold to suggest that precious, painful memories be relegated to that unconscious collective where so many of our personal remembrances stay like little flags strung on the cord of our entire life. But for the sake of my healing, may they flutter there in a carefree fashion, unrecalled, to tickle me well in ways of which I will forever remain unaware.

Chapter 24

It is such a shameful, little panic, scarcely more than a quick intake of breath. How to get rid of this broken deck chair. The dilemma, like dozens of others, represents only the first level of fear. The chair cannot be recycled. I would need a truckload of such items to go to the dumps. Bob is not here to hack it up further to fit in the garbage. I flash on other large objects that will break.

Fears for widows abound in growth, advance in increments, and spread like wild vines. How long can I maintain the deck, the garden, my house, and stay independent? My hip hurts—will I always be able to walk? Will my health last? How long? Or my money? Can I handle the loneliness? Am I loved? How much time do I have? Maybe I have been afraid all my life. I suppose we all are in degrees, especially women who, historically, have been expected to rely on men mostly.

I consider writing about fears since Bob died and at once am seized by frigid bands around my chest and at my throat. Are these barriers for keeping the unruly millions of fears in, or out? Again I retreat quick to Tristine Rainer for help in memoir writing. She tells me: "No matter what your concern—fear of hurting others, fear of humiliating yourself, fear of being judged a poor writer, fear of inaccuracy—there is one piece of advice I give all writers: Write your first draft <u>for your eyes only</u>."

All those "fears" in that paragraph dare me to face the emotional, mental, and physical frights of a lifetime, most of which are related to opening my mouth and getting what I need. What I must do to move forward as a widow is to crack those fears which can otherwise keep me frozen in one place. I can only do so by sharing my truths and <u>NOT</u> <u>keeping them for my eyes only</u>, those honest bits which comprise the purest parts of myself and, therefore, whether they offend or not, the best. Perhaps I have too often spoken words for <u>others' ears only</u>.

Now I feel a pressure on the left side as well, like a scratching at my heart. It seems all my fears wind through a route around my chest and throat blocks, then to the various heart channels for dispersion, dissolution, and, finally, either healthful absorption or successful exit.

If Bob was fearful in his life, he hid the fact. Indeed, he often boasted that he was afraid of only two things: the dark and death. And at his end he overcame those. (Is that how it works, when we conquer all our fears, we die?) For fifty years I was sheltered in the wake of his bravery.

"Don't you need gloves and a shirt and long pants," I yelled one year through the window as, in flip flops and shorts, he attacked the yellow jacket nest between the concrete slab and our house, holding the aerosol can at the crack for the prescribed length of time which seemed an eternity to me. Risk taking hardly phased Bob.

On another day, wearing the same few clothes, he climbed higher and reached further to prune a tree, only to have the ladder collapse, leaving him with scraped bleeding leg and elbow. After determining nothing was broken I saw the humor in his 3-Stooges escapade and made him pose for a picture with his battle wounds, which he did with good nature, though he was not smiling. He accepted the consequences of his fearlessness. But I was always too timid to take a chance.

On still another day I laughed and took more pictures while he, in those same Bermuda shorts, no top, and flip flops yet again gave Judi, donned in her leathers and boots, a push start on her 1969 Sportster motorcycle. There he was, muscular legs propelling him down the middle of our street, bent forward, strong arms pushing hard, small potbelly over the shorts. The snapshot of that is one of my favorites.

As well, Bob was good at volunteering to give people pushes when their cars stalled, as many cars did years ago. We owned two old cars ourselves in those days so we had lots of practice. Bob taught me how to do it. We had a carport, not a garage in the first years of our marriage. I would stand at the front door in the morning, in robe and with coffee and watch him fold his suit jacket and place it on the seat next to him, or hang it on the side hook when there was one.

Hmm, will it start today, I wondered. Maybe he would call, "Okay, I'll push it out to the street," and I would quicken my pace. Gather my robe, grab my keys. After positioning the cars bumper to bumper and putting his into second gear, he would signal me and I would accelerate slowly, then faster, knowing with his precise manipulation of the clutch and gas petals the engine would turn over. Then he waved his arm hard out the window and continued down the street and over to the freeway to work and I returned to the house.

Because it was not uncommon for cars to stall I got as good as Bob at volunteering to push strangers. I always felt confident when I offered. I should remember those tiny risks I took so easily then when I wonder if I can handle my small R.V. alone now. Or when I am frightened wondering what I need and will I be able to get it. Will I be able to open my mouth and say my truth, not "for my eyes only," but for the ears of others? ("Don't ever talk back to your mother!" my father yelled, chasing me at age fifteen, around the Hudson in our garage, brick in hand for emphasis. It was the most scared I remember being.) Can I muster up the energy and determination that I do not possess to demand with authority that which I need from another, at a time when I do not even know if I can exist alone?

It is so much easier to watch through the window when the bees are being killed.

When my proud father boasted about me because I was a good student or a "good" girl, both of whom I was, I appreciate now that he was endeavoring to give me self-confidence in the only way he knew how. "Of course she got all As; she's a Bendinelli, she can do anything." Instead, his bragging set a personal standard for me that I had to be perfect and mistakes were not allowed. I felt compelled to hold that flag high, even as my shaky shoulders ached with its weight. The unidentified feeling I had left me knowing that I would never quite be good enough. Now I know that feeling was fear.

Chapter 25

When I examine my fears as a widow I am back in the playground of my youth, that wide world of cautious adventure, dangerous surprises, and exciting fears. My mother always said that as a toddler I gave away my sand toys. Was it because I was generous? More likely, I was afraid to say no.

I am thinking of the teeter-totter again. The fears that grip widows and widowers fall mostly into two categories, the first of which rests upon one seat of a perfectly balanced see saw, while the second resides at the other end. Those categories of fear comprise the physical versus the emotional. In the early days of widowhood I panicked on this see saw, hitting the ground with a jolt on one end, then holding on tight when flung with abandon into the air. Now I try to maintain a healthy, balanced management of the two fears, but, ironically, in stasis a teeter-totter does not work at all. And there I am, suspended within the lonely space of my new frozen self.

The emotional fears for me have to do with my future. To consider them is to poke a small hole with one finger in a dark cloud to see where the universe ends. I could go crazy. After two years I have accepted the fact that I must concentrate on what I want to do right now, and hopefully this will lead me on the path forward. But still I panic when I glance at the other end of the teeter-totter to where physical fear stays. Will I have enough strength, energy, and good health to sustain life alone?

A study by Dr. Nicholas Christakis at Harvard Medical School has shown that the spouses of sick people face higher risks of illness and death themselves, a phenomenon called the "bereavement effect." The research showed that when sick husbands are hospitalized women are 3% more likely than usual to die on any given day. And if the sick spouse dies, risk of death for the partner jumps five-fold to 21% for men and 17% for women. (I read that after the death of Joan Didion's husband, she never took a walk without carrying her ID.)

I inch away from the eerily balanced see saw. Instead, I climb the ladder of the age-seventy spiral slide. It is good to look around and breathe in the feeling of power at the top. I still felt young when Bob died. The spiral shape may hold surprises at its turns and offer me a smooth ride. But even as I prepare to sit, I remember I will be going fast. I was sixty-nine when Bob got sick. I start down. In 2005 we had been married fifty years, I turned seventy, and Bob died. I am gaining speed now. I fear declining health and overwhelming work. Momentum increases near the next curve. Items fly off the hooks in my brain. I press my leg against the side. I fear loneliness. And lack of intimacy. I am nearing the bottom. I feel old for the first time ever. I cannot see around that last twist, but at the end I know there is discomfort and death.

"You're on borrowed time after seventy," one of Bob's aunts said on her birthday. Now she is ninety with advanced dementia. My mother had Alzheimer's after my father died. It eventually killed her.

Frantically, I shake the sand from between my toes. I stuff my fears and leave the playground fast.

Chapter 26

Bob's father was a determined man, particularly on the road. Before the days of freeways, the state was crisscrossed with two- and three-lane highways, which remained, in my recollection, nearly empty. Tall grasses grew on the sides of these nearly quaint roads with expanses of undeveloped space all around. Burma Shave limericks were on five signs evenly spaced for reading from your black, box-shaped Ford in the 30s and your rounded Dodge of the 40s after running boards had become extinct.

> The wolf
> Is shaved
> So nice and trim
> Red Riding Hood
> Is chasing him
> Burma Shave
> Burma Shave

"We'd go fishing in the backcountry," Bob told me of those early camping trips with his Dad when we first met. "He'd take that old panel truck anywhere!" Bob's dad was a house painter. "Dirt roads, over rocks, jeez!" Nobody had heard of four-wheel drive then. Bob's reminiscing about those trips was not fringed with fear, but with the kind of trust and admiration that a young son might have felt for an example of his dad's stubborn ruthlessness. He would tell these stories at various times: remembering with his brothers at Christmas, over shots of vodka at Russian Easter, or driving with me, the kids in the back of our blue Chevy station wagon loaded for vacation.

"But those three-lane roads took the cake," Bob would say. "He was crazy. He decided the middle lane, you know, the passing one for both directions, was his! And cars would move away quick. At best he would straddle a line. He was never satisfied with one lane." I know this to be true because when I became a part of this family group as a teen, Herm gave me many rides. He did straddle lines, on city streets as well, as if the Russian teen immigrant he had been was by necessity alert always for opportunity.

Perhaps my father-in-law's unflinching "road" work through life contributed to Bob's sense of safety and his apparent lack of fear. I do know that as the years passed I had dreaded being with Bob in the location of a serious emergency involving a stranger, like a drowning or a fire. I became convinced that his courage, combined with his kindness, would oblige him to be the first one to attempt a rescue.

Once, as we waited in a theater line on a downtown San Francisco sidewalk, a drunken man fell and cracked his skull. While the rest of us stared in disbelief, Bob whipped off his new raincoat, which he loved, and placed it under the man's bleeding head. Of course the coat was ruined by the time the paramedics arrived. Without a word Bob dropped the blood-soaked coat into a nearby garbage can. The line was moving then, and we entered the theater.

Also, I know of Bob's fearlessness through the stories people tell. Soon after his death, at the first small gathering of his dearest friends, I heard about a harrowing road adventure they had had once on a steelhead trout fishing trip. Leo, Rich, and Bob, avid fishermen and pals since childhood, had stopped for chili in the town of Willets on the way to the mountains. The cafe had been recommended and the chili, one of Bob's favorite foods, was not to be missed.

"The chili was just the beginning," Leo twinkled in the telling, as the eight of us, three couples and Judi and I, sat around the unlit summer brazier in his pretty patio. We nibbled, sipped, and gazed from time to time into the lush lawn and garden. We were telling "Bob" stories, thank goodness, and we were laughing.

Leo continued, "Bob kept saying 'there's not too many beans, not too many beans, it's good!'" I smiled. I could envision his enthusiastic self leading them into a greasy spoon cafe, eagerly ordering the biggest bowl, breaking saltines into the hot mixture when it arrived. Once he sent to Los Angeles for the Chassen's Chili recipe Elizabeth Taylor and Richard Burton had ordered to the set of an out-of-town movie they were making. "Now this is how chili should be," Bob would announce to me as he cooked a meat-laden caldron for his Super Bowl Sunday parties, or just for himself.

"Oh god," Rich chimed in leaning forward. I knew a hilarious adventure was unfolding. "On the way back he just had to have that chili again." Judi and I, alert, glanced from one storyteller to the other. They were a motor revving up, leaning forward, pointing for emphasis, laughing. Their talk got louder.

"Bob said we could take the logging road instead. We could go *over* instead of around. *Over* the mountain." Rich gestured with his whole arm. I can see Bob in my mind's eye in his usual tank top and shorts, except in 1954 when he was twenty and we were not yet married, tank tops were not worn. He didn't wear shorts then either. Instead, he would be donned in a white tee shirt, a pair of grays, and his high top tennies. Black hair, black horn-rimmed eyeglasses he wore all his life, and never, never a sweater. I can imagine him saying, "yeah, it's a shortcut, guys, we can drop right into Willets."

Leo continued to snigger as Rich talked. It seems they had been rained out, with no fish in the Gualala River. So after one day they had reloaded their camping gear into Bob's yellow Willys Jeepster and high-tailed it towards home. The dirt road Bob talked them into taking was mostly muddy right from the start, and soon, so were they.

"Jeez." Now Leo picks up the story. "Oh, we get stuck all right."

"Yeah, we kept changing drivers," Rich interjects, "to see which one is gonna pull us out each time."

Now they are on a roll.

"We didn't even go that far the first time."

"The wheels kept spinning, remember?"

"We put boards under the tires."

"You try this time, Bob."

"We take out all the camping stuff."

"God, was there mud!"

In the patio the eight of us catch our breath. "Was it the second or third time the road got so narrow?" Rich asks Leo. "All kinds of forks in those roads," he tells us. "Bob wouldn't let us turn around. 'Oh, it's just a little further,' he kept saying. We were covered in mud! You know Bob."

91

Yes, I know Bob never gave up on anything. Nothing scared him. Nothing threatened or deterred him when he had his mind set, whether it was taking a hike with me on an unfamiliar trail—'just one more turn, one more,' he'd say—or finding a new job at age fifty-five after the company he worked for folded. Every morning at eight he left the house in a suit and with his briefcase to make the rounds and check his sources It took him only five weeks to get an even better job. Bob had patience, determination, and best of all, an expectation he would succeed. Of course he would.

Once, when his granddaughter, Sienna, was six and wanted a Batman figure doll, Bob took her shopping. "We'll find one," he assured her as they left the house. After four stores he told us Sienna said, "It's okay, Grandpa. I don't need it." But Bob was on a mission. "We'll get one," I can hear him saying as he dragged the weary and well-loved child in and out of stores like Walgreen's and K-Mart. And of course they did get one.

By now all eight of us in Leo's patio were laughing with relief and release and in solace to one another. Having been together many years, we were bound more tightly even by Bob's death. "But the worst is we couldn't push it out that last time right at the top of the mountain," Rich says. "So we backed it up to the last fork we had passed, which we realized was the right road after all." He paused before quickly adding, "but now the gears were locked."

"My god, what did you do?" Delva, Leo's wife, asked, sounding distressed herself. "Well?" The rest of us—Eddi, Angela, Al, Judi and I—awaited the answer to Del's question.

"Well, we rocked the car," Leo answers. "What could we do? But no luck. The brakes were going out, too, weren't they?" he consults Rich.

"Yeah, and it was getting dark. We didn't know what we were going to do."

In the patio we groan a little. I imagine them muddy and wet and straining to see in a deserted forest that would soon be pitch black. Had I been there I would have been afraid.

"Pretty soon we hear this singing," Rich continues, "and here comes this flatbed lumber truck right smack towards us! There's no way they can get around the jeepster. They stop, get out—big guys—and everybody's kind of looking at the car, saying nothing. That yellow Willys was covered with mud."

"So these guys," Leo takes over, "without saying much, they get two on each side," he gestures picking up something, "and <u>lift</u> the thing, they lift it right up, and turn it completely around. Jeez, they were strong."

"They couldn't get around us otherwise." Rich says.

"They set us on our fork, the one we needed to be on. Bob says, 'I'll drive.' His white tee shirt was really a mess. But you know Bob, hot blooded, no jacket."

"So we finally are heading down the mountain. The brakes don't work, Bob's shifting like mad on only one gear, and we're running out of gas," Rich finishes.

It's dusk now in the patio and we are quiet, with the storytellers remembering, and the rest of us imagining. Where Bob had been brave, I know I would have been petrified. I would have warned, nagged, pleaded. I would have gripped the dashboard, held my breath and, finally, blamed him for all the mistakes. I would not have been laughing as we all had been during the retelling of this adventure. Had Bob been with us he would have been laughing hardest of all with his wicked sense of humor. Of course there was a good chance he <u>was</u> with us, watching and reminiscing, and, if possible in his new ethereal form, laughing.

"Oh," added Rich, as if just recalling a vital fact.

"Oh, yeah," chimed in Leo, who must have been on the same tract. The rest of us perked up in anticipation. "When we finally got to the chili cafe, tired, muddy, hungry, and cranky, the place was closed."

"Oh, no," we groan in unison.

Rich is shaking his head. "When we're walking back to the jeep, Bob is so disappointed he says, 'Somebody else drive.' and he slept all the way home."

Chapter 27

Unlike Bob's dad, my father was a cautious driver, especially on the rutted dirt road leading to our yearly camping spot in northern California. Of course there were no seatbelts on our vacations when I was a child. Had there been my little brother and I would have been buckled up tight in whatever sedan we owned at that time: Ford, Hudson, Studebaker. In the summers between 1938 and 1948 on our camping trips to the bank of the Eel River out of Ukiah we pulled a trailer on two thin tires through eroded roads. The trailer we started with was a small wooden square one, painted green but faded, measuring about five by five and two feet high, a homemade second-hand job. And when that proved to be too small my father went up. That is, he added new wood, never painted, making it five feet high and two-toned. In it he packed our brown canvas umbrella tent, two cots for Bobbie and I, our camp stove, Coleman lantern, his fishing rods, hip boots and tackle box, dishes, pots, food, our clothes, two sleeping bags and assorted pillows and blankets, and, finally, the old metal roll-up bed my folks slept on outside, guarding the tent entrance. After packing the trailer, Dad covered the entire contents with a black tarp tied down along its edge, making a great green and brownish cupcake with a ruffle of licorice frosting.

I never understood why in some years there was no roughly built table at what we considered our private spot near the river down two pot-holed roads, thickly dusted by the summer heat. So we took a card table in case. We washed ourselves and our clothes in the icy river water and we hiked up the hill through poison oak, to which I am allergic, to squat in the bushes.

Nearing our campsite each year, we left the main dirt road and proceeded slowly down the last stretch. That is when I started feeling scared. The eroded, dry, powdery earth created long ditches and deep holes that had a different configuration each year. There were two bad sections on this last half-mile, which seemed much longer to me. The first one was the steepest. I held my breath, my back rigid against the back seat as we began the descent down the hill. That big bulky cupcake bumped along right behind me and at least once I had to turn quick on one knee to make sure it was not hitting us. I always turned back fast because it heaved hard from side to side, now like a bulky baby elephant cupcake just learning to follow in its parent's tracks. My father was quiet, concentrating on the potholes. But it was my mother's nervous energy that set the mood. She braced one hand on the door and the other on the dashboard. She glanced back more than I did, as if jerking her head back and forth would help. Unable to contain her intensity, it escaped as well through her mouth. "Watch out. Oh. There's a big dip."

I was relieved when we reached a plateau where the road was a bit better and level. Then I would glance off to the sides almost wishing we could relinquish our special spot for one of the four or five campsites on either side under the trees. If we could, we would be there now, and safe. But instead my father drove on through the very last section of passage. Advancing in the direction of the river, still bumping along, we would come upon a wide turn and magically we entered enchantment. "Yea," Bobbie and I always yelled then. There it was, our spot on the bank, flat and private, with a shallow, protected eddy from the fast moving river where I spent every day catching poly wogs and where one year I sat for hours with my yellow-jacket stung foot stuck in the medicinal mud.

With that turn I became excited and happy. But like the formidable gatekeeper of a precious fairyland, the last bit slowed up once again. Again the rutted path, the deep powdery dust, the bouncing and swaying of the trailer. Long ago a redwood tree had fallen at the road's end, blocking entrance to our place. It had been cut away, with the huge decaying bulk of it remaining forever to mark the boundary of our paradise. Looking back, I was not afraid of anything else in that wilderness—not the fast river, the poison oak, or the possibility of bears and rattlesnakes. And for two weeks, not the road.

Every morning my father would don his rubber hip boots and we would watch him head either up or down river. My mother relaxed during the day in our private seclusion where the only sounds were glorious blue jays and the constant swish of the swift Eel River. Bobbie and I played all day with no toys. We gathered river stones, tree moss, insects. We collected tadpoles, turtles, and baby lizards that we let go again. In the late afternoon we would hear, "Yoo hoo" in the distance. "Yoo hoo," my mother would answer in a two-syllable sing song call. Then she would gather us up and, walking over river rocks toward him, we all shouted back and forth, "Yoo hoo. Yoo hoo."

Some days my dad did not fish. Then he would wash our hair in turn in the freezing water, holding each of us tight in the current. Or we would go to our "potchy hole" on the other side to swim, crossing upriver where it came only to my thighs, or sometimes daringly on a rope my father strung across the deep part near our camp spot. In later years we all swam across, starting upstream to allow for the drift, plunging in one bold person at a time. (With all those water adventures perhaps I should have turned out to be a braver person. But who knows, maybe I am more courageous than I think.) Then we would walk through a dry meadow, careful of cow flops, to our swim hole, a silty pond on the side of a cliff where all four of us jumped and splashed and yelled with joy.

But at the end of two weeks we faced the scary road again. It was all uphill then, and I was more frightened than before. After everything was packed, with careful roping to secure all our things, my father would start up alone. "Get back, you kids," my worried mother would warn. With both parents nervous I was convinced there was danger. I was relieved to remain at the now bare table a distance away. If I could not see or smell puffs of dust clouding up as the wheels tried to gain traction, if the laboring motor was out of earshot, if I was out of the boundary of my mother's angst, for she stayed closer to the loaded vehicle than we did, if I could be spared the frown on my father's face and the cuss word he may have said, maybe I would not be scared.

We three followed the car in his wake, our shoes making sounds in the dust, plop, plop. We watched him go on the level part until he came to the bad hill. I do not think I ever cried, but the spinning of the wheels when he could not get going frightened me so much I stopped breathing and feeling and thinking. It was as if my life ended each time he slid back, with the trailer jackknifing to the side. Sometimes it took three tries. To distract myself I would look to those safe, flat empty campsites on the side. But the worst was when my father would direct my mother to push the trailer.

"Now you kids stay way over there," she would say. Knowing how nervous she appeared to me when she was in the car, now I thought we would all die for sure. I never needed cautioning to stay way off the road in the dry, scanty weeds. At these times I held my brother's hand tight.

Finally my mother would cry out "Hurray," and I could see he had made it to the top. "Hurray," Bobbie and I called, scrambling through the dust that got in my nose, for now I was breathing again. How quickly the fear left me, as we headed to our traditional powered milk milkshake in Potter Valley to end our trip each year. But the fear returned next summer, and the one after that, and for many years to follow, imprinting upon me a deep pattern of lifelong caution and timidity.

Now I wonder if without Bob I will remain frightened forever.

Chapter 28

Looking back on our lives we cannot believe that we were the main characters there. The settings and actions seem remote. We do not recognize ourselves but for memory. Nevertheless, we are proof of the continuum of time and, most importantly, of the cause and effect connection between all things. I map my life with a line connecting the dot on the dusty hill to that of a nervous teen, then to a worried wife, an anxious mother, a stressed homemaker. The road forked later to over-conscientious college student, writer, teacher. That central personality throughout the journey has influenced my character forever, of course.

Why, with this bird's eye view of my life, would I think I would not be afraid when Bob, my rock, died?

In 1980 I traveled to Oregon for a week-long writers conference. I get restless at seminars and need to make my mid-session escape, which I did then to one of the highest points in the state. I had been directed to a hiking trail that began near the top of a mountain and ended at its peak. So while the other writers took their leisure quietly writing in their tiny rustic rooms or on the broad wooden deck overlooking a rumbling river, I fled in my truck, feeling like a truant racing to freedom. Strange how I always push myself onto the road to wherever the trail leads via the next dot on the map.

Happily, I bumbled along, breathing in the green views and following a local map. The paved road, though narrow, was safe and flat at the beginning. I climbed gradually, still relaxed, smiling, taking it in. Soon, heavily wooded canyons on either side of the road deepened. The climb was gradual, but some miles on, the trees began to thin. That was to be expected, I thought, and all was well, until the paved road ended.

A dirt road. Not a bad one, but a narrow one. No driver continued on unless she was going to the top. Suddenly, I slid from dot to dot back fast to the dusty hilltop of years past. I ordered myself to keep breathing deeply. What had I been thinking coming here? Now the trees were sparse; the shorter mountains around me shrunk down. There was no way to turn around. I had to go forward. As in a nightmare, I sensed it would all come to a bad end. I was on a cliff-side road with a sharp mountain straight up on my right and an equally steep drop (into hell I feared) on my left. Still I advanced. I had no choice. My heart beat hard. I am sure my cheeks were ablaze.

Finally I see the end ahead. I am panting. I am up so high that there are no trees. I glance fast to the left. Hug the right! Ahead, parked cars press against the cliff. The road's end has a tiny turnaround. It'll take two tries for a u-turn. Oh, my god. Braking, backing, maybe flying into oblivion. Perhaps park here first. No, I'll eventually have to do it. I might pass out. My palms are sweaty. Grip the wheel. Go slow. Keep breathing but don't hyperventilate. Thank god for an automatic gearshift. I start turning. I brake. I see nothing but miles of air and distance. This is when I could die. I reverse, back up, slowly, slowly. Do it all again. Oh, my god, I sigh. I made it. I'm shaking.

Looking back and remembering that day, I recall pulling so close to the mountain side of the road as to almost scrap it. I turned off the motor and sat for minutes letting myself return to normal. I was so aware of my tires on solid ground. After a few minutes I could open the door and get out of my truck. I made my way the few steps to the trailhead and then hiked to the top. And though I could then enjoy the view, the hike was anti-climactic after the driving adventure.

In those days I knew nothing of the Tarot. I had not yet met The Fool dancing on the cliff to challenge life. Nor had I met his somewhat more sensible cousin, the Two of Pentacles, carrying his portion of infinity. All I had felt on the cliff then was deep fear, which had traveled along the line of legacy from my youth. I continued following that path from there to Bob's death. Therefore, it is natural that I should be afraid in my grief. But the question I ask myself is this: Might I be able to freeze my fears in place so they may melt away, enabling me to reprogram myself to take risks?

After all, Tristine Rainier says "taking risks in response to fear will become habitual." Though she is referring to writing fears and risks, nevertheless, for me, in writing this memoir of death, the fears in living and in writing are so close as to be the same. Now that I have alongside me on the cliff the outrageous and courageous Fool and his cousin, might my connection to the next dot take a different turn?

Chapter 29

We had been drinking wine for two hours when our hostess instructed us to *hold that thought* as she rushed from the room. We waited.

"Ta Da!" Barb exclaimed in triumph, returning to us and holding a gadget high overhead. She looked like the Statue of Liberty. Indeed, the object was shaped like a torch, with a tapered white metal handle and a round soft-looking white ball, representing the flame, on a cylinder at the top. My friend Linda and I glanced at each other, she with a knowing smirk. I wondered how the others took this.

"Victory!" Barb added, switching the thing to her other hand and resuming the pose on that side. Across the living room the woman named Julie, who appeared to be about sixty, matched Barb's salute with her glass. "Yea!" she added, raising it up high. A younger woman, Deb, sitting near me, tried to do a high-five with Dorothy, a gray-haired lady, who offered her hand for shaking instead. Others giggled from embarrassment or giddiness.

"<u>This</u> is how you take care of yourself," continued Barb, still posing. A long strand of her new red hair had come loose from her bun.

"Right on," cried Deb, who jumped up and posed with her.

"This is what we <u>don't</u> talk about in Group, Barb added, flopping down in her chair, the object collapsed to her lap. For a moment the room quieted. Deb stuck her hand into the back pocket of her tight jeans and eventually returned to her seat as well. Maybe we all wondered just who was nervy enough to pick up on the subject.

⁂

There were six of us that night, as I recall, widows in their first year. Linda attended two grief support groups; that's how she had met Barb. I knew Linda from the first group. The two of them planned this gathering. Bring women in the same boat together, ready to make new friends.

Early in the evening, strange to one another and wearing the proverbial badge of courage over our hearts, we had talked about our lost husbands. Dorothy, who seemed the type to serve on commissions and lead discussions, volunteered that she was really fine. Oh, oh, a red flag I thought. FINE. It stands for Fearful, Insecure, Nervous, Emotional. Poor lady, I knew how she felt. She brushed back her smoothly arranged hair and looked expectant, as if she had called for a quorum.

"I find I'm overwhelmed with maintaining my home, and so tired," Julie said. She did not smile, had a Dutch Boy haircut, and wore a navy blue suit. (Later on she took off her jacket and even untied her bowed blouse, just before she yelled "yea" and raised her glass to Barb.) But now she continued speaking seriously. "I have tried to keep it up, as Jack would have." Others nodded, as did I, for I had been trying all year to prove to myself I could do it all.

The woman sitting next to Julie, whose name I did not get at first—Marian or Mary Ann—was my age, seventy-one. She told us that, and that she had taught Math. "When Felix had been dead only three months a friend asked me what I was planning to do with the house. 'Live in it!' I answered, but the question rattled me. Don't we deserve to stay in our homes without our partners? He had made me think I couldn't handle things alone."

Deb, the high-five woman, was clearly the youngest of us, fifty-ish, with short, spiked hair. "They say keep busy and you won't be lonely," she said. Barb was making the rounds with the wine bottles, red and white. Linda followed her with two plates of cheese, crackers, grapes, carrots, and humus. "Thanks," said Deb, taking cheese. She gulped a swallow of Merlot wine. "I can hardly stand to remain in my house on weekends. I go out every morning to my job. Is that the right kind of busy?"

"Me, too," Linda chimed in, "errands and shopping. I call it retail therapy." She placed the snacks on the end tables, then circled again with the wine. Linda was slim and stylish, with diamond studs in a second pair of earring holes.

More wine, more animation, rosy cheeks. Talk criss-crossed the circle, patterning an invisible Indian dream catcher. Deb slipped her sandals off. Dorothy fanned herself with a paper napkin. When the laughter level rose, I wondered if anyone else besides me noticed we were grieving widows laughing and probably glad for it.

And then we got to dreams.

"Oh, I had a dilly, just last night," Linda said from the middle of the room. She did not know she'd been caught safely in the dream catcher, or that she might tear it apart like a spider web, depending on how good or bad her dream had been.

"I kept telling my father not to leave me." Recalling the dream seemed to agitate her. "I was very young; my parents were putting me somewhere because they couldn't afford me. I guess the Depression." She turned to Barb for confirmation, but Barb just shrugged. "I kept begging him not to abandon me, but the sound wouldn't come out." She stopped talking, crossed to her seat, and took out a tissue. "He ignored me, then vanished. I was still crying when I felt something heavy in one pocket and something soft in the other." Linda blew her nose.

"What was it?" someone ventured.

Taking a deep breath, Linda answered, "A black obsidian stone, smoothed into an oval shape, like a bar of Dove soap—funny, I just remembered, Dove soap has the scent of my mother's cold cream when I was a child.

"Something said to me, 'this stone is resentment; just throw it away.' So I did. In the other pocket was a little heart shaped pillow, torn nearly in half." Linda paused again. "This is weird, but I had the feeling I was being urged to take love and nurturing from wherever I could get it to fix the heart." She had finished talking, and I imagined each of us interpreted Linda's dream in her own way.

Maybe to avert the sadness that began descending upon us again as heavy as Linda's obsidian rock, Deb popped out with, "I dreamed I had sex with a stranger, a good looking one, and it was terrific, even though I felt anxious." She gulped from her glass and added in a wickedly throaty voice, "like I was adulterous or something."

Marian, or Mary Ann, turned back to Linda. "You know your rock dream reminded me of my own rock dream." We shifted to

Marian (I'll call her that), even though we probably all wanted to stay on Deb's lover stranger.

Marian began, "Felix was the foundation of our union, you know, the rock I built on. I could rely on him to be <u>there</u>." She made quote marks in the air for emphasis. "So I could go out into the world while he kept the basics of our lives going.

"So in the dream, I am sitting on a block of cement. It's four-square, very sturdy, but my feet dangle three feet off the ground and I can't get down. When I look around for help I hear a voice. 'You need to get down by yourself.'" With drama, Marian had lowered her voice, and now, returning to her normal tone, she adds, "that was it. I woke up. I guess he meant I'm the one to take care of myself now."

"Amen to that," said Barb, jumping up. "We have got to take care of ourselves. Hold that thought," she said, pointing at us. That's when she rushed from the room.

❦

"My God," tittered Marian, who seemed to have forgotten all about her dream.

"Is that what I think it is?" asked Dorothy reaching for her frameless eyeglasses.

"You bet it is," laughed Barb and nonchalantly set it on the coffee table. All eyes rested on the eighteen-inch instrument of pleasure.

"Well, I figure sex is all over for me," Dorothy blurted out and then covered her mouth, apparently embarrassed.

By now Deb was giggling hard. I could tell she wanted to say something. "What?" we demanded.

"Well, you know what Linda's dream said about her torn heart. *Get love anywhere you can!*" She slapped her leg on the punch line, like a vaudevillian thrilled with her own joke.

"How about EHarmony for dates," Julie blurted out. We were like sorority sisters now. One of the dangling ties of Julie's blouse had been dragged through the humus. "People do find other people on the Net."

"Yeah, if you're thirty," Barb said. "Unless you're a man. Then you can be sixty!"

106

"Yeah, yeah," we all grumped. It felt good getting a little angry.

I thought of my own age, of my posture, more rounded, and of the extra pounds, sagging skin, wrinkles, hair getting gray. Damn those old men running after young girls. Shame on them. The goal nowadays is to be skinnier and younger-looking than ever before in this country's history. And we older women buy into that myth of beauty with nips, tucks, and lifts. Every time we dye our hair to cover gray we say, "young is good." So what does that make old? Who will honor us if we don't respect ourselves as we are? The difference between wanting to look our best and still honor age is a difficult position to maintain. So we accept that looking beautiful means appearing young. Would Barb be just as attractive without her new red hair?

"I want to be Maude," Dorothy murmured. No one responded. "You know, the movie, *Harold and Maude*, where the eighty-year-old quirky but wise and passionate woman is loved by the twenty-year-old boy."

"Ruth Gordon" Julie said, "Hollywood!"

"Dorothy wants a boy toy!" Linda laughed.

"I miss testosterone in my life," Deb said and it perked us up again. "I go to coffeehouses to get near it. Honest to God, and to clubs, you know, bars, with a girl friend."

"The places I go, there is no testosterone," Julie chuckles, "they're too old at the senior center. And I think I'm too old for the barstool." She looks at Deb. "Or maybe not."

"I find myself wondering these days which men use Viagra." Barb left us with that provocative thought and went to make coffee. It was getting late; I guess we were winding down.

"I've got a confession," Linda half whispered.

"Oh, good." We hunkered in.

"I got a massage the other day. Usually I get a woman, but my regular wasn't there. Well, this guy was about forty-five, strong, and best of all healthy looking. I was so horny when he began the massage I wanted to jump him right then. I didn't dare move. By the time I left I was a jittery mess. Never again a male."

"You know what you need." Barb called from the kitchen. Again, all eyes went to the coffee table.

"My friend told me the third year is the worst," I said. Not just sex, but for intimacy and loneliness. By the third year she had created a new normal, but within it, the reality of her husband's absence deepened making her feel even lonelier."

I am sure they were thinking, as I was, that three years is too long a time to feel such loss, such longing. Another widowed friend once told me she wanted a male companion, not for sex, but for an escort. A pal, a pair, a hand to hold, someone to walk in with, a body for balance at dinner at a restaurant.

Maybe that is what we really crave in a male partner now. A cuddle, a touch, an intimate talk with the opposite sex again, regardless of the degree of male hormone he has in his body. Perhaps that is all we want.

Or, maybe it's not.

Linda called the day after the gathering. "I just have to tell you the dream I had last night." She sounded more agitated than excited. "Well, I met this man and had some sort of visit, lots of talk, fun. Suddenly he wanted more. He wanted sex, but he wanted closeness, or something. It was all vague. I told him I didn't feel that way about him." She paused, maybe thinking of her husband, Bill.

"So, what happened," I asked. "Is there more?"

"Well, then the dream shifted and I was having the same kind of fun with a young Asian woman, long black hair. And I suddenly wanted more. This is embarrassing, because I'm not a lesbian, but she said she just wanted to be friends."

I think I answered Linda with something like "wow." I could hear her take a deep breath. "What do you think it means?" she asked finally.

"Well," I began slowly, "besides all the other grieving stuff you are going through, it looks like you have even more choices to make." I didn't really know Linda that well. I think that's all I said to her, but throughout the day I found myself remembering her dream.

By afternoon, resting with a beer in the backyard near my pool I was wondering how people will come in and flow out of our lives now. Some we will want to keep and some we will lose again, and how will that feel each time? I took a sip of cold ale and allowed my glance to drift with the pool ripples. Do we work hard at connecting here and there adventurously, or do we just flow with the current, resting momentarily in our own lonely—or not so lonely—small eddies. Maybe we should not choose at all, but just tread water and wait.

Or, again, maybe not.

Chapter 30

Solitude, a somber word I have loved, no longer offers solace, for without Bob to intervene, solitude becomes loneliness. During my extended solitude now, I ask myself what I may be learning from Bob's death. I hear him saying again, "Life is an adventure to be lived, not a lesson to learn." Ram Das wrote, "Be here now." And the Laughing Buddha is no fool.

So, with the "L" word cooing in my ear, like a mourning dove sad and low, I listen to Buddha and Bob and try to laugh through the adventure of life. And I heed Ram Das to observe how I feel at this now moment. Still, I do believe in the mandatory lessons as well, connecting the stops on my life map to create a line by which I may continue to drive forward.

On certain days, for months after Bob's death—from my moaning, groaning cocoon, doubled over and rolled into a sealed enclosure, rocking and releasing, crying until snot poured out freely and I did not care—I begged his forgiveness. Forgiveness for any time in our lives when I hurt him, or expected too much of him, or pushed too hard, or made him sad, or dumped on him my own fears, dissatisfactions, doubts, mistrusts, suspicions, and weaknesses, or when I ever may have misjudged his wisdom, his strength, his character, and his abilities.

> 1970
> I lighten my load at your expense.
> How selfish of me, how small to give you half
> so I suffer less. Why don't I carry it all?
> Because I'm afraid, so I run to you,
> but another pressure begins anew—
> the weight of guilt at having made you suffer too.

I told Bob over and over I forgave him for anything he may have done or thought he had done to make me unhappy. I assured him we both knew we forgave each other. Nevertheless, I continued to beg. It saddened Bob always to see me sad. So, I also implored him not to be upset in his other world when he saw me left here crying on earth. Strange how in my loneliness I always begged for forgiveness, as if all my transgressions against him may have caused him to die.

From Bob's death, then, I learned forgiveness. I would be gentler with others and with myself. Small grievances matter little. I consider family behavior and that of friends, and I dismiss everything. In fact, nothing much matters at all. Or rather, ironically, everything is important and yet nothing is important. "It is what it is," Bob was fond of saying. And now I believe him. Maybe forgiving and being forgiven assuages loneliness.

In an area of high earthquake occurrences I have ignored earthquake preparedness for my home, but if the third year of grieving is the worst for loneliness, as my friend warns, I had better ready myself for the upcoming jolt to my heart. If I believe that we grieve in the manner in which we have lived, and I hold this to be true, then how did I handle loneliness through my life, I wonder?

I flash on 36th Avenue in San Mateo where my father built a home for us when I was fifteen.

"Do I <u>have</u> to help this weekend?" I would whine, anticipating another boring time as a go-for in the hot sun. I would hand tools to my father all day as I watched him soaking and dripping with sweat for which he took salt pills. Months later when we moved in, I was yanked out of my old school, not for the first time. Worse yet, I was forced to leave my Foolish Five friends behind, a group of inseparable and corny girls. We had sewed big polka-dotted, red and white skirts with matching bows for our hair. "Everybody, don't forget, we're all wearing them tomorrow," we would announce to each other on certain days.

Upon moving, my parents promptly bought a grocery store and worked every day until dinnertime. After school I was in lonely charge of my brother who was four years younger than I. Also, I cooked dinner for everyone. Four o'clock in the afternoon was the hardest.

What I remember of loneliness was not how I felt personally—I never identified those feelings; perhaps I would not have stoically survived if I had—but rather I remember the feel of the environment. I can see it: a still living room painted cream-color, wall to wall beige carpeting, everything very clean, blond modern furniture, a glass-top coffee table, built-in book shelves with no books, quiet, large front window facing a quiet, empty suburban street on a hill. I can never see me there, but I sense myself seeing the room. The environment was lonely all afternoon, and I was part of the environment.

But I knew none of this then. My parents worked hard and were tired. I worked hard at school, did homework, covered for my brother, and started the dinner at the correct hour. I did no extra curricular school activities.

"You made too much salad again," my father said to me occasionally. A plain red kitchen with a chrome dinette set, Dad at his place, Mom taking over the cooking, I think. I believe we were between dogs and before parakeets, so there was a glaring absence of movement throughout the house. The salad consisted of boring head lettuce and tomatoes, oil and vinegar. I had peeled and prepared the potatoes earlier. I am pretty sure it was mostly me who cleaned the kitchen alone after dinner.

"It's starting!"

"I'm coming," Mom would answer and appear from upstairs with her little cigarette can of bobby pins. My mother put pin curls in her hair every night while we all watched our 1950 black and white television set. But the program was over early, and there was nothing more for me to do but ascend the empty stairway to my quiet, still room.

I withstood those days of loneliness. But how did I?

I think there were two conditions that got me through. The first was an unconscious resiliency created by having attended four grammar schools, a junior high, and two high schools. And, most pertinently, I had parents who worked hard, were hard on themselves, and expected no less from me.

One simply went forth.

My saving grace was Bob. He had become my boyfriend at my old high school. "But Cornelia..." is the only line that I remember from the school play we were in together when we met. It was his line and I was Cornelia. Bob, who was first, as was I, in the birth order of his siblings, was steadfast and determined. He was not giving up his Cornelia. Each week, after I moved to San Mateo, he trudged up the hill from his Daly City home to the Mission Street Greyhound. Fifteen miles later he walked a long six blocks to my house on 36th Avenue, only to turn around when he had called for me. Then, together we sauntered back the distance to the "show", which is what we called the movies in those days.

On the way back to my house after the film we always stopped in the dark grammar school yard between two buildings to kiss, not once, but many times. This was the delicious, innocent highlight of the week for us both, the wedge against loneliness for me.

"The week dragged by," Bob might say in a hushed, hoarse voice.

"I miss you so much," I would whisper to him, just as I tell his picture now.

We took the last block home slowly. Our moment was nearly over. At my front door, after a farewell kiss and a reluctant release of hands, Bob would retrace his arduous trip back to Daly City.

My oasis in the desert of the 36th Avenue neighborhood, Bob, is gone now. I suppose I must simply go forth. But with a very big difference. I was a girl then. After a lifetime of learning about feelings, in this bout of loneliness I am able to identify my feeling of desperation as the debilitating condition that it is. I understand the consequences of the unchecked cancer of loneliness. The responsibility to cure myself is up to me. Am I better or worse off with more knowledge? And though our cancers are different, I recall I did not do well in curing the one Bob had.

Bob wanted to be cremated, with his ashes scattered in the Delta, which he loved and where he kept his boat. In the Fall of 2005, three months after his death, on a crisp day in his favorite season, Autumn, I drove to Antioch with Judi in the passenger's seat lovingly holding the box that contained Bob's remains. Prior to that day of clear blue sky and pure white clouds, the harbor master had kindly consented to drive Bob's boat, the Beboka, for me.

114

1967
I can't think of anything cozier
than us four in a little enclosure
bobbing in the bay on a lovely clear day.
If we catch t'will be great. Bob'll cook 'em.
Either he, Suz, or Jude will have hooked 'em.
Then after some family discussion we'll just drift,
read our books, and have luncheon.
Oh come Sunday how happy I'll be
with my family out on the sea.

The harbormaster took us in a slow circle near the Antioch Bridge, in a spot at which Bob had often fished. The sun glistened like fish scales on the calm water. Judi stood a few feet from me as, crying the whole time, I poured Bob's remains in an even path and watched them descend to a gentle repose. "Ah," is what I felt Bob sigh, "at last and finally, the cool water my body so thirsted for near its death."

A water sign, a Cancer, Bob was at home then, and both Judi and I fully sensed it. But now nothing remained of his physical self; I had no special place to sit and visit with him. Of course I would continue to talk to his pictures throughout the house. I would still curl up to his side in our bed with tearful memories in the dark hours. But, still, there was no marked place, like a tombstone at which I might visit him.

I, too, am a water sign, a Pisces, a little fish who has never had her fill of swimming.

1975   *A Valentine for Bob*
I bought a white bowl at St. Vincent de Paul
'cuz a crab and fish are glazed inside.
Blue Cancer, Pisces Pink, corny I think
after twenty years wed. But we'll share it alike
and I'm glad that delights me.

I believe our astrological signs heavily influenced us from the start, for we had swimming pools nearly the whole of our married life. Vinyl ones. First, when our daughters were small, a round above-ground one, three feet deep, with a ladder for climbing up and over.

"Watch me, Mom," my daughters would take turns calling, their hair in pony tails, maybe wearing nose clips. Five strokes took them across. Thirty years ago in a different house, with the help of the neighborhood boys, Bob dug out a hole for a full-sized pool, half in the ground, half above, with a wood deck built up around each end. By then our girls were teenagers. Every spring we opened the swim season. Bob and I fixed up the yard: planting flowers and veggies, hanging wind chimes and decorations, placing beach chairs, vacuuming the pool, stoking up the heater, and awakening the water from its winter sleep.

Throughout its glorious history our back-yard pool witnessed many visits, including ten years of family Fourth of July swim parties, with the young nieces and nephews and, finally, with their children. In time the festivities waned in size and number and that felt right. Our daughters moved on, the families enlarged and scattered, and our friends got older and less water frisky.

Then came a renaissance of laughter and fun-filled years with our granddaughters from Alaska for the annual summer visit with their mother, our Star.

"Three more sleeps!" Terra might giggle over the phone when she was tiny.

"How much ice cream did you get this year?" Sienna might ask. "Mommy!" I could hear her call, "they've got fifteen half gallons!"

Bob worked hard readying the space for his precious girls, including the inflating of about twenty-five pool toys, colorful bits of large and small plastic that bobbed and floated and provided hiding places in our exuberant games of water tag. There were alligators, seals, two small canoes, rafts, rings, snakes, and balls. We had two versions of Samu, the mother whale and her baby, complete with sweet eyelashes painted on. When Baby Samu got a hole in her, Terra cried.

"It's okay," comforted Sienna. Of course, their beloved Grandpa came to the rescue by patching it.

"Where are you taking your granddaughters this year?" our friends asked.

"They never want to go anywhere," we would answer. Truly, the swimming pool at the Edna Way Resort, as they came to call our home, was the centerpiece for these visits.

The pool is in the backyard area, hidden from the patio, which is more public. Gradually, the back became an even more private space. Only the crab and the fish continued to use the pool. I did daily laps and Bob floated around in the meditative, relaxing way that suited his character perfectly. After work he would set his vodka gimlet on the edge, and, as if in slow motion, take leisurely strokes, gaze at the trees, and let the workday stresses melt away. I did not swim at this hour. Rather, I brought a glass of wine to my favorite chair there, wearing a visor against the setting sun. We did not talk. I watched him unwind, saw his strong shoulders and smooth skin moving above the surface, quietly, powerfully, as peaceful and wise as an ancient sea turtle. He might hold on to a pool toy—we still blew up two or three—and just drift.

Throughout the history of the pool, Bob and I, the water babies, were the constants. When we swam together my favorite memory is of draping over his strong back, my head nestled into his neck as he slowly walked the deep end. Water. Nurturing. Deep peace. Bob.

The last summer the granddaughters came was the one when Bob died. For these two years since then I have used the pool alone. At first that felt lonely. I would sit on the secluded deck and cry. I spoke aloud to Bob.

> 1980 *Conversation*
> "Would you grieve me if I died?"
> "Why?"
> "Would you miss me at all?"
> "Do you feel like excess baggage,
> not missed, not called for?"
> "No," he says, but I think he lies.
> So I try to tell it right
> "I seldom long for people gone,
> I'd go on living in the now—
> and be lonely for you all my life."

After a few weeks I began to revere that pool space as the private shrine it had become. One day I realized that this was the place, like a cemetery plot, where I could visit Bob. Surely his spirit was there. I bought a small angel statue and stopped sharing the backyard with people altogether. I was healing as I swam back and forth. I called this sacred place my Meditation and Healing Pool. I invite friends to my patio; I welcome them to my house. But most people do not know about my back yard area, and that is the way I leave it.

Being near the pool comforts me. Hypnotically, I gaze at the four items that float in patterns created by the pool filter flow and the breeze. I may be resting or sipping a beer, getting ready to swim or simply owning my spiritual space with Bob. I hear the variety of chimes singing from the tree branches and my house. The hanging mobiles have history, like the brightly painted fish one from a family trip to Mexico. Sometimes I am sad. Mostly I am at peace there.

The four objects in the pool consist of a blue raft patterned with tiny, brown monkeys, a small purple swim ring, a yellow sun with rays, whose painted face sports sunglasses, a happy smile, and even curly eyelashes. The last item is made of hard plastic—a blue and white chlorine-tab container.

"Get out of my way," I yelled many times when it bumped me on my head during laps. I bawled it out so often I felt we were on a personal basis, so he was the first one to be named. There is a Tom Hanks movie, *Cast Away*, in which he is lost at sea and so lonely he befriends the basketball, his only companion in the raft. He personifies the ball with its brand name—Wilson. So I, too, named the basketball-sized chlorine container Wilson. After all, I felt lost at sea and lonely also. It followed I should name the others.

Chuck, the monkey raft, all brawn and no guile, is sometimes in my way but always there to serve. I can't get mad at him; I need him for support. "Yah, Chuck, just get out of the water so I can do my laps," I mumble coming up under him and heaving him onto the deck. Brian is the brains. Small and discrete, he is somewhat sneaky. "<u>Now</u> where are you?" I ask when I want to squeeze my head and shoulders through his argumentative self so I may float suspended and relaxed. Sunshine is just that—bright and bobbing. "You make me happy," I tell her. "You remind me to play." Wilson is the hardheaded boss, always greedily plunging into the filter intake box, apparently anxious to push ahead in the world and take care of necessary business, as I am.

The pathos of my pool scenario reminds me how lonely I am. But the humor in the situation encourages me to laugh. One day last week, after I had swum and replaced the solar cover, I noticed Sunshine stuck under the ladder. Still smiling bravely and wearing her saucy sunglasses, nevertheless, she was flailing frantically from side to side, caught in a jetty stream from which there was no escape. Had it been Chuck stuck I would said, "that's like you, hitting your head against the wall." Brian would have masterminded a way out. Wilson pushes too hard against the filter opening, so he needs to be restrained.

But that stoic smile on Sunshine's face as she kept going forth, only to find herself unable to be free, made me cry. Over a yellow inflatable pool toy I cried! So I lifted her out. "It's not so bad Sweetie," I said setting her free to move outward into an uncovered area. "Look at the rest of them; they're all pinned under the cover. Now they are just blue bumps." She floated out slowly, still smiling.

After watching a while, I turned away from the pool, from Sunshine, and from another day. And I returned to the house to continue to go forth.

Chapter 31

Recently, I took coffee to bed one morning, first time since Bob got sick and died. Sipping and gazing out the window, I saw a squirrel run along the patio fence, as always. A storm had broken the fence, leaving it brutally detached with a gaping vulnerability to the world next door. The squirrel came to the end of the leaning fence and stopped short, like an exercise in quick freeze. She didn't want to change course and continue on the ground. She wanted to complete her regular morning route to the backyard. She needed her familiar path. The gap in the broken fence was too unfamiliar, too wide, too dangerous to make the leap and go on. She paused, looked down, stared ahead at the disruption, stayed still, then retreated.

I drank some cold coffee and cried a bit. I relied on that squirrel to be able to do her familiar run. I thought she would be able to jump easily. Of course she can, I flashed, just before she ran away. Squirrels scurry, bridge, persevere, and fly through the air to other places. Their little legs slip on wet wires but with strength and determination they carry on scampering, nesting, burying food, guarding home. Only once ever did I see one fall from our pine tree, lay stunned, jump up fast, rush into the swimming pool, (from which I quickly skimmed her out with the net), and run back up the tree.

The squirrel on my broken fence had not sprung forward, but I did, from my bed, to see how wide the space was—two feet. She could have made it easily, but her morning pattern had been abruptly changed and she had been shocked. I knew she would find another route, perhaps through the branches of the lemon or olive trees along the fence. Maybe across the roof. Possibly a better route after all.

Nevertheless, I felt impatient then to have the fence fixed fast to show her that things will be comfortable for her again soon. At that moment of panicky feeling I wanted her to know that too. I wanted her to be okay in the world, and of course she will be. How could she not?

I turned from thoughts of the squirrel, deciding to reread my journal entries since Bob's death two years ago on July 14, 2005. I wanted to see how I was doing. With my life so disrupted it is hard to believe I will be all right in the world alone. Perhaps I would see a pattern in the writings to encourage me, some secrets I had hidden for myself, like peanuts buried in the ground, to restore my joy and delight.

January 26, 2006. I'm restless. I keep asking myself what I'll do with the rest of my life, which now feels like someone else's. I realize it's the same question I asked myself when I was twenty!

January 30, 2006. After the death of a spouse we rediscover who we are, they say, and if we're lucky, why?

February 1, 2006. I stop reading the newspaper this morning and pull my journal towards me. Just read that they have finally discovered why married people live longer. Because the touch in holding a partner's hand releases endorphins in the brain that confront stress. So I visualized holding Bob's hand again and it worked. I felt something, a sensation in the heart and stomach area. Oh, a good feeling. I will practice remembering how his hand felt when we'd take off in a plane. Always we would hold hands then, as a totem for safety. I will do this often.

The cat's on my lap, cradled in her favorite baby position, purring hard, both of us warm from the reading lamp just over my shoulder. With closed eyes, she has melted like hot cheese in a sandwich between my robed arm and chest. I relinquish Bob's hand for now and imagine Dorothy is holding me instead. I close my eyes and picture myself in her position. How nurturing—no wonder she's lived to eighteen years. I feel soft, warm, restful, supported, safe, protected.

Suddenly, I see myself in the swimming pool with Bob. I am draped across his back again, held, supported, safe, protected, as he walks in silence through the deep end of the warm water, my front to his strong back, my legs wound around his stomach, head resting gently aside his.

I cry a little then, and Dorothy decides to get off my lap. Did I want to "get down" off Bob's back when I had had my current fill of love? Yes, there was a moment when we both knew it was time to move on to the next moment of life, perhaps to attend to the pool, maybe to prepare dinner.

When Dorothy left, I slipped into Bob's hand again and remembered its perfect fit: large, warm, clinging tightly. "Oh, too hard," I'd say at times through the fifty years, and he would ease up. I will continue to hold hands with Bob and look for that surge that runs from my hand to my heart, that combination of sadness, ecstasy, tears. When it overwhelms me after awhile I will climb down from the current fill of Bob's love.

February 4, 2006. I see where widow Coretta King died, seventy-eight years old. She had it all—heart, cancer, stroke. Am I waiting for one of those?

February 6, 2006. Saw a video on graceful aging: "Green Winter." It seems that many worldwide countrywomen who live near mountains, walking up and down them, live to 106 to 114. Now I look at all the extra physical work I need to do without Bob as adding to, rather than taking from, my life. I will make the steep hills of San Francisco my mountains.

February 10, 2006. "My Bob" I keep whispering aloud when I am alone.

March 8, 2006. Sometimes I feel the wound is scabbing over but without a drain tube.

March 10, 2006. I saw the light at 4 a.m. Very dark. In bed. Couldn't sleep. So I meditated.

"My body is my guide. I am an earthly creature guiding myself in this physical plane. I follow my body on this earth. I am guided. I am filled with energy."

Saying all this made me feel like I was having an epiphany and I found myself laughing and crying all at once.

That's when I saw the light.

There was a bright flash through the drapes. Not like a car passing. It was sudden, pure, and silent. Lightening had filled the room. I waited for the thunder to follow, or rain. Nothing but absolute silence. I knew then it was a sign congratulating me on my self-discovery. If, instead of a light, there had been words, they would have been: "Yes, you're right. You see the light!".

Is this a kind of "going crazy" I hear about with widows?

<u>March 23, 2006</u>. All I have now is everyone.

<u>March 30, 2006</u>. I swear my right hand looks more like Bob's all the time. Since I started visualizing holding hands with him, this hand has taken on the wider shape of his. I always have seen my mother's hands in mine—smallish, well formed, strong but slender. Maybe it's the extra work I am doing physically. No, I think imagination and visualization and yearning have caused my hand to change.

<u>April 1, 2006</u>. I've noticed some adult children have a biological time clock which is different from the earlier one about procreation. This second one goes off when one parent dies. It jangles the son or daughter awake abruptly and from that day on he or she views the remaining parent through a cockeyed hourglass. The distortion renders the mother or father misshapen, frail, needy, and slightly imbecilic. With one parent gone, the remaining one appears suddenly to be very old. (My goodness, look, she's stiff upon rising, she has wrinkles, she takes a nap! When is her driver's license renewable?) And then the parent must be on guard against the self-fulfilling prophecy, even if she still rides horses, cuts down trees, or goes out dancing.

Convinced we need "looking after," which may or generally may not be true, subtly the kids begin for themselves the long, mentally arduous, noble responsibility of "burden-ship." The feel of the parent draped across one's shoulders is at first hardly noticeable to the child, just a gentle pressure like a nagging tickle of a feather. But as the years drag on, although the parent does indeed become physically more frail, she, paradoxically, becomes heavier and the adult child shifts position, now very much aware of needing to readjust the load she carries.

I'm convinced the alarm goes off prematurely in most cases. Sometimes it is ticked off by the old people. They believe children take care of parents, and why not start now? They may ask kids to fulfill their needs when they are still capable of running their own lives. After all, they rationalize, "we can afford to take a breather." But they don't realize, I believe, how expensive that luxury is. A therapist told my friend (and she told me) to find someone else other than her children to talk to in her vulnerable, grieving state. That was my own wake-up call.

Not that we widows and widowers do not or should not rely on our families for support. We are all there for each other emotionally, physically, mentally, and spiritually. That is how it should be. But I will not sound an alarm which awakens my daughters with a jolt to a sense of "frail-mother responsibility." Only if and when it becomes absolutely necessary should we widows do that.

In all fairness to my girls, they are aware of the situation. Recently Judi said to me, "I decided I am not going to treat you as if you are old and feeble. You are capable." That showed me she was turning off the alarm clock herself. Now, I have got to admit a little help now and then is appreciated. Nevertheless, I applaud her attitude, for her sake <u>and</u> for mine. But mostly for mine.

<u>April 18, 2006</u>. I feel like I'm drowning yet know how to swim.

<u>April 24, 2006</u>. Do people die, not because they become old, but because they have said goodbye so many times by then?

<u>April 25, 2006</u>. Giving Bob's bike away was harder than I thought it would be. I think of him riding around by himself. He never announced he was going for a ride or talked about where he went. I think I never asked him. Pity. Although he probably wouldn't have answered much. "Just around." When I donated the bike, I took off the lock-up chain and the little cloth bike basket. Although my similar basket has remained empty, his was stuffed full with things I doubt he ever used. These items are so dear to me I cry as I list them: Bicycle tube, key for the chain, zinc oxide that he wore

like clown lips, bicycle patch rubber cement, a second tube (I guess for me when we rode together), a "Save your Life" glow clip flashing reflector, a tire air gauge, a skinny wrench, two other wrench gadgets, a set of midget wrenches never out of the case (probably a gift from one of his girls; graciously he always said "thank you, that comes in handy"; never did he utter, "I have a million wrenches" or fishing flies, or hats, or handkerchiefs.)

May 5, 2006. After Bob died I panicked at the thought of fixing things that broke. Now, ten months later, I find myself saying, "oh well, I'll have to fix it."

May 31, 2006. When I am watching the movie of myself, a living creature now in the community of the world, existing side by side with millions of others—doing work, playing, talking, planning, just living—when I watch this movie I feel fine. For I have always done these things, mostly on my own, even as my beloved Bob was there somewhere.

Then I switch to the movie of Bob-no-longer-exists-and-I-will-never-see-him-again, and I feel devastated.

Switching to a third film, my future, I feel vague and bewildered and forever striving to clear a space to just be, preferably in some creative, peaceful persona.

So, why do I change channels? Though we need to face our grief, is it really necessary to stick a needle in our wound in order to heal? When I focus on me now, a healthy, vibrant human, and not compare my life with the past and Bob or with the future and old-age frailty, I am well. I can go on. I can be.

In grieving, then, I will mostly remember to switch to the channel of the movie of me now.

June 23, 2006. Coming up to a year. To now I have been 1) diligently taking care of business to prove to myself I can; 2) seeing friends and attending two support groups; 3) writing; 4) spending time with Judi, as she is at my house half of each week—this has been emotional support for us both.

<u>June 24, 2006</u>. There is a mound in the middle of my king-size bed. But I never climb over. I stay in my safe little nest each night. I don't know if that makes me happy or sad. I have another nest in my cozy kitchen booth. It has been my seat forever. These days there is a small crack in the vinyl where I sit, like a new life beginning to hatch.

<u>July 14, 2006</u>. It is one year today since Bob died. This is the hump I've been moving towards. I needed to go through all the seasons of the year without him, each a sad beginning. I feel no different. What will the second year bring? Today I will vacuum the swimming pool as Bob always did. I see him moving the pole slowly, meditatively, silently. It would take him a long time to do this chore and I wonder what he was thinking, gazing into the pool, staring deep into the substance he so loved—water.

<u>August 1, 2006</u>. We sat in a circle on the floor. "Women in Transition." Early on, when I had heard most of them complain about their lousy husbands, I thought, "what the hell am I doing here?" Anxious to get away, I stood quickly at the end. By then I was pissed. A woman made one last remark and I said loudly, "My husband would never do that! I would give anything to have him back. I'm happy he graced my life for fifty years. He was a great man." Dead silence. I crossed to the front door fast, and before making my getaway, I added, "You are great women. Life positively. Life is good." I was outta there!

Driving home, I was glad I had shown anger instead of stuffing it. All evening I had wanted to say, "pull yourself up, dry your eyes, and smile." I got an interesting new view of myself through this encounter. We all struggle through life as creatures genetically programmed to do so, and what for? Comes down to: *go with the tide with maybe a tiny sail up for direction.*

<u>November 11, 2006</u>. I am divinely guided.
I am spiritually protected.
I am universally nurtured.
I am personally motivated.

January 1, 2007. Took my coffee to the driveway with my little chair, hoping for a New Year's sunrise. Just missed it; sky was getting gray, then suddenly a second sunrise! All bright and orange again. A second chance. What a sign.

January 31, 2007. Having a hard time deciding how much of my life to keep, how much to change, and which is best to do.

March 1, 2007. Not writing here as often. Taking Prozac less. But watching lousy TV movies more.

March 8, 2007. Grieving is harder as time passes, not easier. Why? I think because Bob is gone longer now.

May 7, 2007. I am weaned off Prozac completely after two and a half years. I have cried more than usual these past three months since stopping.

June 1, 2007. When does my new life start? I think when the new and old finally dovetail to form an indecipherable seam. But when is that?

July 19, 2007. Four p.m. The saddest part of the day. It feels like there is no one anywhere. Quiet. I miss my dead people. What do others do at four p.m.? The same—they finish the day. How do they feel? Maybe I should ask them. Maybe that's the origin of the cocktail hour—a four to six p.m. depression.

Chapter 32

Doctors, therapists, grief support members, and savvy friends continue to ask me, "How are you sleeping?" Avoiding depression means getting enough sleep. But as with all the issues of widowhood grief, there is a delicate balance to be maintained: If I go to bed too early I awake in the night to two hours of a double life. My mind gropes in the dark for the real me somewhere in the background, with events and people protruding in rich detail. At the same time, in my current existence, I remain at the surface of this waking nightmare where I toss and turn searching for depth and meaning.

In desperation I scour the confusing picture of my present, restless life, which is so similar to pictures in the "Magic Eye" books. On those pages the viewer studies a nonsensical pattern long enough for the eye to play a trick. Magically, a scene appears, perhaps of a unicorn in a forest or a clipper ship at sea. Then one steps from a flat jumble into a sanctuary of multi-dimensional existence. With relief and pleasure I study every leaf and bush of this comforting place. I want to step behind the familiar unicorn, sink down into the ground, and stay.

My real life is there.

But my eyes soon refocus and I am again staring at a cluttered pattern, which I recognize to be the mid-night nightmare of my current life.

When a psychic asked if Bob came to me in my dreams I answered "not often." Later I scanned my journal with curiosity and was surprised at the pattern I discovered. First of all, I saw that seven months had passed since his death before I dreamed of him at all. In that first dream in February, 2006, Bob had one week to live. And I, therefore, had only one week to say everything. Bob appeared quiet and solemn in his hospital bed at home. It was not clear he knew he was dying. In a foggy state of extreme anxiety and sadness I sensed I was able to say all that was needed.

The dream was a metaphor because in real life in those desperate days of that time I was living under the same pressure and anxiety to accept Bob was truly gone and to do all I needed to do to stay sane.

One month later I saw Bob again faintly, but only his face, like the wizard of oz, omnificent. Still not smiling. Upon awakening I knew he had been watching over me those past months. I worried that his passage from life to death may have been difficult and made more troublesome by my own grief.

And then in the ninth month after his death, March, the month of my birth, I had two river dreams. "What shall I do on my birthday?" I asked myself in the dream. I was wearing a dress of a bright, jumbled pattern and a chaotic print jacket that clashed. At the riverbank I took myself in my arms for the baptism. "But this is going to be a death, not a birth," I said. "I will not be reborn; instead I am putting myself to death on this day of birth."

I woke up fast, thinking, "River Styx." But I was not crossing over; I was flowing down. Still, the purpose there was to die, unlike that of the previous week's river dream. In that river dream, the first one, I was sitting in a dark gray rubber tire tube floating down the ripples, laughing. A thin rubber drainage tube of the same color hung out from my heart and over the side. I awoke smiling. Dying, birthing—actually, I am not sure which I was doing in either dream.

When Bob returned to my dreams the following month, April, he was smiling, finally. My impression was that he had decided it was time to place himself closer. Whereas past dreams featured only his face hiding, almost like a Where's Waldo puzzle, now he willingly floated towards me with a lightness of spirit. His body heat surrounded me like a cloak.

A week prior to this dream I had made arrangements to scatter his ashes in the Delta, as he had requested. And two days after the dream he was happily swimming with the fishes.

Two months later, in June, with summer coming on and so many bodies advertising the fact in television commercials, Bob's peaceful self swam towards me again. A school of human bodies,

130

diaphanous, vague, vaporous, each with Bob's bright face swirled around me. Coarse and fine particles drifting through Delta waters. I saw a progression of Bob's faces, like snapshots through the years: laughing youth, proud father, serious adult, obedient son, now the quiet smile as if he knew something special, then the wise look, and, finally, resignation and no smile. Had an angel whispered to him that he would die early?

At last Bob seemed at peace. Of course, I was still far from it. I had passed Joan Didion's magical first year of grieving, which did not mean a thing. Though I could not yet scream, I felt no anger. I continued to pine for Bob, dismiss his faults, praise his strengths, and, in general, deify him.

I began analyzing the purpose of Bob's appearances in my dreams. Looking back I realized that at first he held silent and distant vigil for me. He did not smile; he was having his own difficult time very possibly. Perhaps he watched me on the River Styx, dying and birthing and landing with a laugh. At that same time I released Bob to his own watery wish. He smiled; in dreams he seemed again his happy self.

In the dreams to come in the last trimester of this nine-month dream cycle, I discovered Bob pushed me along in my grieving work. "It makes me sad to see you so sad," he may have whispered, which he said to me in life. He helped me by presenting himself as less than perfect the next time he appeared.

On September 29, 2006, I woke up because I could not breathe. In the dream I am cuddled close to Bob on the couch, holding his arm and speaking quietly into his ear. "I love you so much. If I ever hurt you I didn't mean to." I whisper on and on. I do not want the girls, Star and Judi, who are sitting on his other side, to hear me. I am trying so hard to secretly convince him of how much he means to me. But he continues to talk to the girls, his back to me. "I can't hear you," he calls over his shoulder, "that's my bad ear." I try to reposition myself but I can't let the girls hear me because they will say I am mean to Dad. "You are always so mean to him!" But he keeps talking to our daughters and I wake up crying and gasping for air.

And, finally, at the end of the nine-month period of dreams, like untying the rope that held his boat in the Delta harbor, he cut the ethereal cord. I awake furious. Finally I feel rage. I dreamed he had a girl child with another woman. Bob is bragging. "Isn't she adorable!" The child is Asian. A-sin.

I began to wonder what secrets Bob may have had in life? Did he love me as much as I loved him? Why should I feel guilty that I may not have treated him well enough? Was he always able to give me what I needed? He even carelessly neglected to mention he had a cell phone until he wrote it in our address book. Hey, I was beginning to appoint him to idol status. Bullocks! That had to stop, for both our sakes.

After having recorded that dream of anger in my journal I noticed I wrote: *I love him. He wasn't a saint. He's gone. I'm alive. I'm free to get on with my life.* Nevertheless, though I am now unmoored and by necessity outward bound, I will always miss the best person I ever knew. Thank you, Bob, for this hard birth, or maybe I should say "miscarriage," for the resulting separation is not at all a blessed event.

Chapter 33

On June 27, 2005, seventeen days before Bob died, he said to me, "I had better get into my wheelchair soon."

I was feeding him breakfast as usual, a few mouthfuls of cream of wheat. The summer sun shone into our bedroom through the patio window. Bob did not realize that now he was bed ridden. From the straight-backed chair I sat upon very close to his hospital bed I withheld the next bite and then answered him.

"Honey, you won't be using your wheelchair anymore." I wanted to cry. I waited.

"That's it? I'm just going to stay here until I die?"

"What do you think?"

He was silent for a bit, staring ahead out the window. "I guess that's the facts of life," he finally answered with what sounded like resignation, though I had never known him to give up on anything before. This conversation felt too important to be real.

I put the tray aside. "Do you want to talk about anything?" If he said yes I would know he had accepted 'the facts of life.' But I was hoping for no.

"No," he answered, then added, "when the girls go on their trip." Star and the girls had been here off and on for a few weeks. They would be in to say good morning soon. I lowered his bed, helped him turn on his side, and sat very close on my adjoining twin bed, my arm resting on his through the slats.

"Where do I die? Here?" He was facing me but I don't recall he was looking at me.

"Yes. I will be with you, or Judi, the whole time." Judi had spent hours just sitting and watching him sleep. "Are you afraid?"

"No. I am in denial. And I don't want to talk about it more now."

I think he closed his eyes. With my hand pressed firmly on his bare arm, I wanted to reassure him. "Judi and me will be here," I repeated. And then this strong-willed man, determined to perpetuate the normalcy of life as he knew it, corrected my grammar.

"Judi and I," he said.

Bob's last birthday was two days later on June 29. People sent balloons. The girls made a cake and a book, "Seventy-Two Reasons Why We Love You." The teens acted jolly, Star put up an energetic front, and I could not bear to let down. In the snapshots we took, only Judi's face reflected the gloominess of the occasion. Bob's weak, thin, sad face smiled faintly in one picture. I gave him a gold watch with a dial that could light up at night. But now he was too weak to push the knob.

On July 4, 2005, Bob finally relinquished hope. In the afternoon he had a dream that he was paralyzed. "No, you are just weak," I said, lying down on his bed with him.

"I'm not healthy," he said.

"No," I agreed and waited. He asked a lot of questions then, like what is the "schedule" and the "plan." I told him he was in charge.

"If I had a gun I would be in charge," he answered sharply. He wanted to know the "process" and where they were taking him. I said they were not taking him anywhere, that he was in charge and could leave anytime he was ready.

"But don't they expedite it?"

"No, no." My poor darling. I never dreamed he was thinking that.

"Then what was that paper I signed?"

"Not what you are thinking," I said. "You are in charge."

"But how do I do it?"

"Just go to sleep when you are ready."

He slept then and awoke asking me, "do you think a person can have just one stroke?"

After that, in his conscientious manner, he checked with me each time he awoke. Through morphine dreams he would whisper in the night, "am I dead yet?"

"No, my darling, you are still here with me. Wake me whenever you need me."

We had put a bell by his bed for summoning us when his voice became weak, a large, loud brass one Judi bought him. I donated a heavy, gold costume jewelry necklace and we hung it on the wheelchair in the days prior when we had pushed him and the chained bell from room to room.

Now, faintly, he said, "Where's the b...?"

"The pill?" I asked.

"The ..bb.."

I moved closer. "The bill?"

"The BELL!" he shouted with force. Where did all his unbelievable strength come from?

Bob's sleep became agitated so he needed more morphine. Sometimes he would awake confused. One day he got angry. "You told me it was up to me. Well I keep going to sleep and I keep waking up. Will you tell me when I'm dead?"

"Yes, I will tell you, "I answered.

"Okay," he said and fell back asleep.

I had purchased a tape called "Peaceful Dying." After having listened to it first, I decided it was one I believed he could hear. Delicately I had asked him, and when he consented to listen I brought in his portable tape player.

"Nice," he said as it played soothing music and words. He listened to it several times after that.

The next day I asked Bob if I was keeping him here with my love.

"Yes. Let me go."

I let him go as I stroked his thick, wavy gray hair.

"Thank you," he said. He listened to the tape again, mumbling that he should be going, the tape says to go.

A time before that day Bob dreamed a group of people came and told him he had ten days left. His daughters and I wondered if he was thinking of the hospice people who appeared and left. Or was there a morphine-induced dream? Maybe Bob had had a vision of angels. The ten-day period came and went. We discovered his angels had given him two extra days. During that time, with renewed determination, he tried to get out of bed. I had sides put up on the bottom end then, for he would have fallen had I not entered the room in time.

On the following afternoon as Bob and I remained together and listened to the girls in the backyard swimming pool, he said, "I want to be out there with them." It broke my heart.

"I know you do."

"I love you very much," he says.

"I love you very much, too," I answer.

"I love Sienna and Terra," he adds. I nod.

He mumbles something. "Are you saying Star and Judi?" I lean in. He smiles at me.

"They love you, too." I say. And then he sleeps again.

In the two-day grace period the angels had granted Bob, he talked some more. He instructed me on practical matters, asked me to write letters after his death to certain people he loved and told me to take good care of the children. ("They are good kids"). He said his only regret was that he would not have more time with me.

The house was quiet in the evening of July 14, 2005. Terra was watching television. Star was on the phone. Sienna had returned to Alaska already. Judi was at work. Bob and I were alone in our bedroom. I put on "Peaceful Dying" and lay down next to him. He slept peacefully on his back. The words invited Bob to let go, to feel peace, to relax, and to know his life had been good. There were interims of music between the words, an angelic melody, which I hummed along with until the next gentle words came forth. Finally the tape finished. I sat up, leaned close, and watched every one of his even, gentle breaths, the inhalation of which he held a moment before releasing.

I took up where the tape left off. I told Bob about his life. I told him how much he was loved. I encouraged him to let go. Then I sang the melody to him, which I followed with more words about him, his life, our life together. I never took my eyes from his face because I had a strong feeling that one of the next even breaths would be his last.

And then it was.

With the last breath, his mouth, which had been slightly open, closed. His lips softened. His whole face had the peaceful expression of his well self. Had he been able to speak he would have said, wisely, "Ah, yes, finally I understand." As I observed that amazing split second, I felt he was smiling. I believe that in that moment he abandoned his body, that body I so loved and for which he had no more need. (Indeed, when Star entered the room soon after she saw a vision of him looking down at his corporeal body, with his arms extended overhead in a Fred Flintstone victory pose. "Yabba dabba doo, I made it!" she felt him say.)

I covered Bob's hands with my own and kept talking and talking to him about his life, and more. I cannot remember all I said. It was a privilege and an honor to have shared a life with this man. Sobbing, my face wet, I could not stop talking to him. Twenty minutes passed, or a lifetime. And, finally, when I felt it was the right time, I walked away to tell the others he had passed on.

Chapter 34

"The substance of grief is not imaginary. It's as real
as rope or the absence of air, and like both of these things
it can kill. My body understood there was no safe place
for me to be."

Barbara Kingsolver
The Poisonwood Bible

Night. Walking home fast down the middle of the street. Keep looking back for figures. Street deserted. Panting. Fourteen years old. Not safe alone in the night world, parents warned. Never safe there.

Younger still. At a friend's house across town. "Sure," her mother says, "but be back at nine." Cool twelve-year-olds. Dressed in style: men's grays worn low and white shirts with sleeves rolled up. Strolling in the dark. Down the main street. People, shops, lights, more people. But it's wrong alone. Ought to be home. In my own home. Not safe out in the world alone. Scared.

Ouch! Forehead against heavy glass door. A rumbling rattle. Glass not broken. Eyeglasses did not break. Forehead not bleeding. Check. Brain on the rain. Must put a warning decal. Back in the house. Break down crying. No "oh, Honey, are you okay?" Drip, drip, drip. The fireplace continues to leak. Had stitches been needed...a heart attack...a stroke...or a fall off the ladder...how far away is the phone? "Oh, Honey, are you okay?" Can't stop crying, alone. No fire in the fireplace for so long. Fire not safe alone.

Rain, rain, more rain. Drain the pool. Electric pump. Overflowing filter box. Drip, splash, drip, splash. Electric pump in the rain. Concentrate: Step One, Step Two, then and then only plug it in. Must stay safe alone.

Decisions alone, eat alone, television alone, scared alone. Mind always thinking, solving alone. Sleeping alone in a new small bed.

Abandoned. He left. He went. He disappeared. He's gone, forever. Vacant. Vacuum. Loss. Replacement? No, never. No replacement ever.

Big house, single resident, quiet neighborhood. Out the window, widows. Walk and talk. Stooped further forward each year. Their houses needy. Hip aches, eyes fade, hairs thin. Withdraw from the window. Shrink back abandoned. Alone. Declining in the dented, nested couch. Never again.

Body understands there is no safe place for me to be.

Chapter 35

When people ask me about Bob's illness I answer, "He was well; he was sick; he was dead." That is what the shock of it all felt like. He had been an active, healthy seventy-one-year-old man when the first blatant, fatal symptom of cancer appeared. Nine months later he was gone. I also tell people it took nine months for him to be born and nine months for him to die. The nine-month dream period in which he first appeared to me smiling and ended with him giving me release was another cycle of natural and spiritual significance.

I had thought that once I had passed all the seasons of the year without him there would be relief from my anguish. Stoically I accepted autumn first, Bob's favorite season, with its crisp, cool days, which he relished without sweaters, wearing only tee shirts. Then I embraced the winter holidays determined to reach for that sparkling star of joy. In the spring I readied our pool and planted our garden, thankful for being surrounded by nature that cradled me for crying. Summer offered warmth and healing alone in my backyard. Like a mirror, my mind reflected the message from my brain: The first magical year has passed, now carry on. But I felt no better.

It was only when I noticed the metaphysical presence of cycles of nine and reflected upon them that I experienced relief from body-racking grief. My awareness of the cycles comforted me. Their occurrence gave me permission to acknowledge the vast mystery that exists beyond my realm of conscious knowledge. I believe there is a large picture, like a sky map, from which I cannot stand far enough away to see completely, a pattern of overlapping cycles mystically twinkling on and off, like a universe with a sense of humor. I follow the path of one of the celestial cycles for a time, then pick up the rhythm of another, trying not to control the journey too closely. I try to be the Tarot Fool, adventurous and brave, and not remain frozen and closed to the guiding signs. The cycles of nine help me.

Recently I asked Judi, who is a numerologist, about the significance of the number nine. Without pause she answered, "Nine is the highest number on the spectrum. It represents all knowing, all seeing. Key words are <u>compassion</u> and <u>forgiveness</u>. It means caring for all of humanity."

I think I answered "wow."

Judi went on. "Nine has to do with universal love and letting go. When you've worked through all your karma, all the numbers, you might not come back again." While I was relating this information to my feelings about the nine cycles, she added quietly, "Dad was a Nine."

This conversation took place on the phone. "Are you still there, Mom?" Though it is true I could not yet scream aloud my rage and frustration, at that moment I had achieved a different kind of release. I had felt myself melting a little, letting go, stepping back from my mind, back from the cycles, my peripheral vision enlarged. My sky map took on a few more stars.

In the first months after Bob's death, when I had feared I may not be able to exist without him and therefore moved with haste to prove to myself I could, I bought chairs.

(Of course I also tackled more tangible projects to keep myself grounded. I had the house and country cottage painted, repaired the dry rot, installed a new drain pipe, replaced a fence, had the roof treated, slaved over the swimming pool upkeep, planted a garden, painted the decks and patio furniture, replaced a heating system, sold the RV and Bob's boat, and bought a new bed finally, which was the hardest chore of all.)

The chairs were an incidental happening. The first one I bought was a brown armchair for the living room, replacing a shabby one. I purchased it on a whim, had it carried to my truck, and wondered how I could possibly get it into the house. In retrospect, I see I was testing myself. Though I felt alone in my neighborhood, I stretched myself to compose a mental list of what turned out to be nine (that number!) men I knew in adjoining streets that I could have turned to for help. I needed to know that, because I felt I had no network of support.

The next chair became four. Maintaining my house meant upgrading the patio. I got a new glass top table and four metal chairs. They were followed by two new white resin ones imprinted with roses. Soon, at a church yard sale, an adorable little antique replica caught my eye. Now, I should say that some people consider my house to be cluttered. I admit I am a gatherer. There is so much in the world to love and bring home. I am never so happy as when I am gathering. I told that once to Bob after years of his eye rolling when I entered the door with armfuls of dried branches from my walks. It was the first time he really heard what I said about my gathering, and he never objected again. Now I think my gathering of things and people helps me to replace. I weave across my loss to mend a net, to cause a connection, to create support.

Having observed widows and widowers in their quiet but frantic desperation, I detect a repeating pattern of attitude and behavior that I call Holey Net Dystrophy. We strong people afflicted with this malady complain of having no network of support. Most of us have histories of taking good care of ourselves. We are competent and able. With stoic determination we self-sufficient folks have persevered through life, inadvertently creating scenarios of perfectionism through the years. It seems no one can do anything as well as we can. So no one tries. When we lose our partners people expect us to grieve well, which we mostly do throughout our healing process. By then, though, we have forgotten how to ask for help. Maybe we never learned how to do so. Or were refused too many times. Perhaps we do not even know we need help. The outcome for us needy, strong souls is that in our sad mourning we feel we are completely without support. Blinded by our frightening inability to replace our great loss we cannot see the large holes in our nets that need mending.

So I continue to gather. But I do like order. Therefore, my clutter is orderly with everything in its place—shells, rocks, gems, bric-a-brac, and larger items like three couches, stereo, televisions, computer, a couple of large plants. I do not need chairs, but I bought the darling antique replica anyway. The last chair was for a desk in Bob's room, a place in which he kept his souvenirs of a lifetime, his own collection of dozens of small gifts displayed on shelves he mounted after his retirement.

My friends and family laughed, "Another chair?" I kept seeing other ones I liked but finally I reprimanded myself. Enough is enough. Why such a fixation on chairs, I wondered. They caught my eye in thrift stores and yard sales. I luxuriated in deep-cushioned ones in department stores, sinking down with comfort to watch the passing shoppers. Once I had a patio party and when the guests had departed I took my glass of wine from chair to chair, feeling the view from each spot and recalling the afternoon as the sun lowered and the glow of the festivity continued to energize me.

I have loved parties my whole life. I like giving them; I like attending them. As a child I would become thrilled to nervous exhaustion at my birthday parties. When I was seven, and wearing a rose-colored jumper my mother had made for the occasion, I was so excited awaiting guests to hand out the favors—small, clear glass replicas of early telephones filled with tiny ball candies—that I ran a fever, was put to bed, and missed it all.

In our house in Daly City my father build a knotty-pine rumpus room in the basement, complete with bar and stools, a piano, a phonograph, and an old nickel slot machine in one corner. We had parties! As innocent pre-teens, my friends and I played the old 78 records, danced the jitterbug, laughed, took pictures showing boys in bowties and girls wearing party dresses with ruffles, ate homemade birthday cake, drank coca cola, Nehi orange, and Hires root beer from bottles and used one of the empties for our daring games of "Spin the Bottle."

During my teens and after Bob had entered my life and been there for a year, my parents planned a move from Daly City to San Mateo. One late Saturday afternoon, weeks before the move, Bob picked me up from my job at a Colma floral shop.

"Let's go to the beach for awhile," he suggested. In those days the kids hung out at Thornton Beach on the ocean side of Westlake behind Daly City.

"It's not very sunny," I said. Daly City is known for its fog, especially in the summer. It seemed strange he was suggesting this, but I was up for anything Bob planned. Well, it was freezing as we huddled on our blanket. I'm not sure but I think we were the only ones there. The fog blocked the horizon, and finally we could only <u>hear</u> the water. My hair was dripping.

"I guess we had better go," Bob said glancing at his watch. When we got to my house my mother instructed me to go downstairs and see something. As soon as I opened the door to the basement and started down the carpeted, darkish stairway with Bob following, I knew what was happening. A wave of warmth washed up those stairs at once. More than warm though, this air was electric.

"What's going on?" I feigned. I felt excited descending through the shadows; I think the main light was off in the basement.

"I don't know," Bob played along as we made our way to the closed rumpus room door. We groped through dimness. I turned the door handle.

"Surprise!" We stepped into bright light and color and noisy energy. A crowd of kids held a butcher-paper banner that reached from wall to wall. In big, uneven letters of various colors the words read, GOODBYE, BEV. WE WILL MISS YOU! Have we ever been nurtured more than by our childhood friends? How we clung to one another for encouragement and support. How would we survive without people? I still have that banner.

The best parties I ever gave took place in our tiny apartment on 18th Street in San Francisco in the early years of our marriage. It was so crowded we often spilled into the outer hallway.

"Come on in," someone sitting on the hall stairs might say to another tenant returning home. There were three other apartments occupied by three widows. We were the youngsters. They all loved Bob, particularly Lovey, our arthritic landlady for whom Bob polished the brass mailboxes each Saturday.

At Christmas time one year I borrowed my mother's large carnival-glass punch bowl which had belonged to her mother (and now to me) and in which my father always made his famous eggnog. Yolks beat with powered sugar, whipped whites folded into rich cream and whole milk generously laced with bourbon and brandy.

"I'll bring one up to Lovey when they're ready, before anyone gets here," Bob called from the bathroom where he was finishing the Brill Cream touches on his then dark brown hair and studying himself in the mirror for one last moment.

"Okay," I answered in the kitchen and brought out the ingredients. I wore a cute ruffled 1950s Christmas apron as I seriously and efficiently prepared the first bowl. Guests arrived, men in red bowties, women with jingle bell earrings or corsages of small, plastic poinsettias. Our three tiny rooms filled quickly.

I made the second bowl of eggnog amidst lots of laughter and rosy cheeks. On either the third or fourth bowl I was having trouble focusing. When I cracked the first egg I completely missed that large punch bowl. There it lay on the Formica kitchen table, a big, golden, accusing eye staring up at me.

"Oops! Oh, oh," came from a chorus of friends watching. Lots more laughter.

"What's up?" Others poked in to see. We all thought this was hilarious, especially me. I missed again, twice, and we roared. Often I have thought that that was the best party Bob and I ever gave. And it was not because of the eggnog. Rather, it was all that glorious intimacy. Why did I thrive so on the electric charge that played its private game of tag from one of us to the next?

I am as happy at large parties as I was in our little apartment. I love cocktail parties with their small talk and opportunity for anonymity and observation. Though I crave intimacy, I thrive in an impersonal atmosphere like that of the huge, pulsating New York party in the movie, "Midnight Cowboy." There, I can flow or dance from place to person, communicating, touching, at once being a part of a pattern of people that, like mercury, evolves fast to yet another configuration. There is a tinge of the metaphysical in such a gathering of humankind.

Once, years ago, a need forced me to plan an impromptu party two days before Thanksgiving. Even though I worked full time and was a college student again with a class that very night, I was frantic for that party. Crazy. Bob played host and I was the last one to arrive. I loved the feeling, like a secret, of walking into the vital energy of a group of people together talking, eating, moving from room to room and watching them connect. Friends from Berkeley brought strangers and after a while one man asked me, "so, how do you know the people giving this party?"

"I live here. I'm one of them." I laughed. I have often wondered why that incident tickled me so. I think it was because I had loved creating a small, fleeting community of people who may or

146

may not have known each other prior but who were willing to cling together.

The memorial celebration of Bob's life was the grandest gathering I ever arranged. When I hugged each of the hundred people I clung to them, not only to stay grounded, but also to assure myself I was still connected to this world within a pattern of other people. And then in January, six months later, to the possible chagrin of some who may have thought it was too early, I gave a party and had the cake decorated to read, "Happy Birthday to Us All in 2006." I did it to celebrate life and our links to one another.

One day a friend came for coffee and we giggled together over my chair-buying binge. We had been sitting in the kitchen. For some reason I sat in Bob's place that day, not in my own usual spot on the cozy curved nook. As she made ready to leave she quipped, "Have fun buying chairs."

"Oh, I'm definitely finished with that." I said, hugging her good-bye. When I returned to my lukewarm coffee at Bob's place I was still smiling about the chairs, recalling them in order and counting as I went. When had I decided enough was enough, and why?

I counted...seven, eight, nine. Oh, my god, I thought. I had stopped buying last month. I ticked off the months on my fingers. The figures corresponded to Bob's having been gone for nine months. Nine months after he died I stopped bringing chairs into our home. Astounded, I realized I had averaged a chair a month for the magical, mystical number of nine months.

I replaced my cup in the saucer, let the tears flow, and wiped my face with a paper napkin. The thought came to me that although I cannot have my Bob with me here anymore, I am determined to survive.

There is a watery place in my mind to which I go to be with Bob. It is neither my backyard pool nor the Delta, which is his body's resting-place. At this special place I sit on a beach chair with my feet in the sand. Sometimes I wear a filmy, burgundy dress I loved once. It flows when I dance, like angel hair in the breeze. Mostly though, I go as I am when I close my eyes, glancing in my daydream to the chair next to mine. Bob sits there peacefully, with that sweet, little smile he gives me. We hold hands that rest on the arms of our chairs pulled together, and in between loving looks at one another we watch the ocean. The crab and the fish together again.

One day there recently I felt lonely despite Bob next to me. The wide stretch of beach was empty. So I brought in my friends. With the vast ocean as background they appeared one by one and in groups, all facing me. The ones I see most often and those I have known all my life stood closest. That's not many, I thought. I need my dead people, too. So I called in my mother and father, dear friends, old pets, relatives and acquaintances. They extended towards the water in staggered placement. They all faced me, they all smiled. Now, that was better.

But then a strange thing happened. More faces appeared behind my people, down the beach all the way to the water line. And when I let go of Bob's hand to stand and get a better look, a little sob caught in my chest. For, as far as I could see into the ocean and towards the horizon there were people hovering and looking back at me. People I did not know. But what I did know was that they could be mine also. All I had to do was go to them. I remembered one of my favorite books then, *The Art of Loving*, in which Erich Fromm, the author and prominent psychologist, said that to know someone is to love that person.

To this day, two and a half years have passed since Bob's death occurred. At the beginning of this New Year my horoscope stated information with uncanny perception regarding the past. *"The big pattern indicates that you have worked extremely hard since the year 2005 but that you are now entering a new stage of life."*

Recently, I read about Deepak Chopra's "Ten Keys of Happiness." I was delighted to see that the first key relates to a belief regarding our human bodies, a belief that I have long held myself. Key No. 1 states: "Listen to your body and eavesdrop on the mind of the universe."

Definitely, I will continue to listen to my body, for it is my guide. But I will remain aware of other bodies around me as well. I most assuredly will stay connected to people. Of course I will. I have the chairs to prove it.

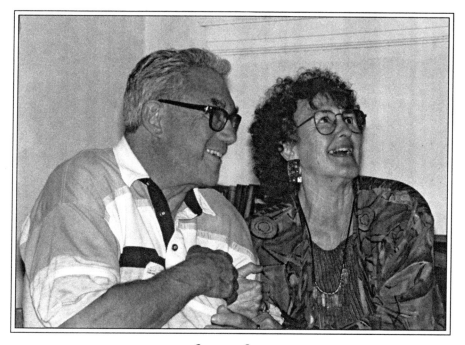

Bob and Bev
2000

9 781935 125402